FIRST RESPONDER'S GUIDE TO ABNORMAL PSYCHOLOGY

Applications for Police, Firefighters and Rescue Personnel

T0181267

FIRST RESPONDER'S GUIDE TO ABNORMAL PSYCHOLOGY

Applications for Police, Firefighters and Rescue Personnel

William I. Dorfman
Nova Southeastern University
Fort Lauderdale, Florida, USA

and

Lenore E.A. Walker
Nova Southeastern University
Fort Lauderdale, Florida, USA

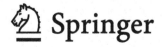 Springer

William I. Dorfman
Center for Psychological Studies
3301 College Avenue
Nova Southeastern Uniersity
Ft. Lauderdale, Florida 33314
e-mail: dorfman@nova.edu

Lenore E. A. Walker
Center for Psychological Studies
3301 College Avenue
Nova Southeastern Uniersity
Ft. Lauderdale, Florida 33314
e-mail: drlenorewalker@aol.com

Library of Congress Control Number: 2006929449

ISBN-10: 0-387-35139-6   e-ISBN-10: 0-387-35465-4
ISBN-13: 978-0-387-35139-1   e-ISBN-13: 978-0-387-35465-1

Printed on acid-free paper.

9 8 7 6 5 4 3 2 1

springer.com

TO

Phyllis, Karen, Aaron, Will, Zack and Eric

Karen & Steven, Max, Benjamin, and Oliver; Michael & Roberta,
Micaela and Maya, Sara, Laura & Andrew,
Jacob, Anne, and Jonathan

AND TO

All the *First Responders* who make their world a safer
place in which to live

Table of Contents

Introduction

The devastating events of September 11, 2001 crystallized in the national consciousness the critical role of our police, firefighters and emergency medical personnel in dealing with emotional as well as physical trauma. These *First Responders* played central roles in addressing the overwhelming medical and psychological needs of massive numbers of victims and brought continuous attention to these dedicated public servants over a period of several months. As a result of this crisis, our country has developed a renewed appreciation for the contributions these First Responders make on a daily basis. In particular, we have come to appreciate more fully the important functions these personnel serve in evaluating and intervening with individuals suffering from chronic psychological and psychiatric impairments as well as traumatic stress resulting from accidents, domestic violence, natural disasters and other life threatening emergencies—all in addition to the more highly publicized disaster. While the psychological literature supporting the educational and training needs of emergency personnel is voluminous, there is relatively little published that is geared to the needs of First Responders covering the range of psychiatric and psychological disorders with which they must deal. We have written *First Responder's Guide to Abnormal Psychology* to address their needs and those of students who aspire to fill those roles.

First Responders, personnel who are often first on the scene when an emergency occurs, are police officers on their daily beat, detectives trying to solve a murder case, firefighters responding to a conflagration, or air marshals protecting passengers on a flight. They are transportation safety workers, probation officers, FBI agents seeking to identify terrorists, detention center staff, wardens and deputy workers in our jails and prisons as well as military police keeping order after a bomb explodes. Few of these individuals will have had training in understanding people's emotional responses to stress and trauma or the signs and symptoms of psychological illness. We have written this book to address these critical issues.

The book has been organized so that professors who are teaching courses in criminal justice, psychology, social work, or emergency services can easily adapt material to their syllabi. We offer current information in clinical and forensic psychology, as well as crisis and trauma theory employing real life examples of the principles discussed in the text, and concise tables summarizing the cardinal features of the various mental disorders that First Responders encounter. We have chosen to eliminate references to research literature in the text that are so common in traditional psychology textbooks written for professional mental health workers or psychology majors. Rather, we have attempted to enhance readability by emphasizing the clinical and practical nature of the issues we describe, adding source material at the end of each chapter for those who wish to explore any topic more fully.

The text includes chapters covering the major psychological and psychiatric impairments, including cognitive disorders; schizophrenia; depression and bipolar disorder; anxiety, somatoform, and dissociative disorders; substance use disorders and personality disorders. Another chapter summarizes the most relevant information on disorders common in children and adolescents including discussions of child abuse, domestic violence, and juvenile justice. Finally, specialized chapters address crisis, terrorism and trauma theories, and intervention strategies useful for First Responders, in addition to the role of therapeutic justice that includes sections on drug, mental health and domestic violence courts, involuntary commitment, and the insanity defense.

The National Institute of Mental Health reported in 2006 that mental disorders are the leading cause of disability in the United States and Canada for ages 15 to 44, with an estimated 26.2% of Americans these ages and older—about one in four adults—suffering from a diagnosable mental disorder in a given year. The Department of Justice claims that over 60% of all inmates in jails and prisons in the United States have experienced a mental illness at some time of their lives. We hope that our book will enable our readers to perform their critical jobs more effectively, more sensitively, and with a fuller appreciation of the very debilitating role stress, trauma, and mental illness play in he lives of citizens they serve.

We want to express our appreciation to our editors especially Sharon Panulla at Springer for their support and patience as we developed this text. We offer very special thanks to Dr. Rosemary Timoney who carefully reviewed and edited preliminary drafts of the manuscript. Our text became more readable under her thoughtful and sensitive direction.

WILLIAM I. DORFMAN
LENORE E.A. WALKER
Ft. Lauderdale, FL
January 2007

CHAPTER 1

The Role and Importance of First Responders in Dealing with Psychologically Disordered Individuals

WHO ARE FIRST RESPONDERS?

The term *"first responders"* became publicized during the aftermath of the terrorist attack on the World Trade Towers and Pentagon on September 11, 2001. First Responders are trained persons who respond to an emergency or crisis call. They may be police officers, fire fighters, emergency medical technicians, mental health counselors and psychologists, medical staff and doctors, crime scene technicians, child protective services workers, security guards, first-line soldiers in combat, and in some cases, office managers and school teachers.

First Responders rarely know what they will find when answering a call. Police are trained to intervene in a home invasion but if either the perpetrator or the victim has a mental health problem, his or her behavior may well be unpredictable, putting everyone in danger. Firefighters are trained to save a burning building, but how to persuade a mentally ill person that it is safe to leave may require another set of skills. A child protective services worker may have to make a home visit in a building being "guarded" by a paranoid schizophrenic who sees the worker as the enemy. Security guards may find disheveled and disorientated people, but may have no training in how to deal with them.

We all became aware of the firefighters who lost their lives on September 11 in NYC when, unaware that the buildings were about to collapse, they ran into the World Trade Towers to save people trapped inside. Many New Yorkers became First Responders that day, trying to help their friends, family, or even strangers standing next to them deal with the magnitude of the tragedy that unfolded before them. Strangers talked to each other, trying to make sense out of what had just transpired. Stories of heroes that day emerged; the woman train dispatcher who stopped the NJ Transit trains from going towards the station under the World Trade buildings, the office workers who helped colleagues down the stairs when they became afraid to continue, the people in the

1

fourth airplane destined for the White House who went down with the plane rather than comply with the hijackers' demands, and other brave people just like them. The Red Cross sent hundreds of volunteers to the scene over the next several months. Many learned that providing a listening ear, a blanket, and warm cup of cocoa was critically important. Later, psychologists and other mental health workers provided crisis counseling for these First Responders to prevent them from developing more serious trauma reactions themselves.

We learned during this mass catastrophe what others who were trained to respond in an emergency knew when they first arrived at a disaster scene; caring people make a difference in saving lives and preventing further psychological injuries. But what about those whose mental status is not very stable even before tragedy strikes? Or those whose mental illness seems to propel them into the criminal justice system repeatedly? In the following chapters, we attempt to explain what we know about mental illness both before an emergency strikes as well as afterwards. We will describe the impact of crisis situations on individuals; how the brain and nervous system control human behavior; and how mental health professionals use their skills to diagnose, evaluate and treat psychological dysfunction. We believe that First Responders need this knowledge in order to deal more effectively with patients and victims who may suffer both physical and psychological trauma (Box 1.1).

WHAT KINDS OF PEOPLE WILL FIRST RESPONDERS DEAL WITH?

Trauma Victims

The first responder who answers a crisis call may find people who are traumatized by the current situation or those who were mentally ill previously and then became retraumatized by what they had just experienced. Again, September 11 provides good examples. Many people who observed the planes hit the buildings, watched people jumping out windows to their death, climbed down smoke-filled staircases to save their own lives or watched the buildings collapse in front of their own eyes developed acute and chronic traumatic stress reactions. Some of them developed the more chronic *Post Traumatic Stress Disorder (PTSD)*. Many who watched the images on television over and over again were traumatized. Those who lost family and close friends in the buildings also developed these reactions. Police and fire-fighters developed traumatic stress as well. In some cases, these reactions lasted for months and years afterwards. Others were shaken by the experience but moved on with their lives, rarely showing any emotional impact. What was it that motivated people to respond in such widely different ways to the same experience?

BOX 1.1

Other Victims of 9/11: Therapists, Social Workers

By Alison McCook

NEW YORK (Reuters Health)—Social workers who counseled large numbers of patients traumatized by the September 11 attacks in New York appear to be at risk of developing the same nightmares and flashbacks as their patients, a new study reports.

Study author Dr. Joseph A. Boscarino explained that this phenomenon, known as secondary trauma, likely results when therapists or social workers hear descriptions of traumatic events from patients, then picture those events and become traumatized themselves.

"As a therapist, you can be at risk from treating these people," he said.

However, he noted that social workers who said they had a supportive work environment—meaning, for instance, that their boss was sensitive to their needs, or they received a lot of time off to de-stress—appeared to be protected from secondary trauma.

For social workers and other therapists who have already developed secondary trauma, "there's every reason to believe they should have counseling themselves," Boscarino noted. "Just like a victim who directly experienced (the trauma)."

In an interview, Boscarino, who is based at the New York Academy of Medicine in New York City, explained that previous research has shown that spouses and therapists of Vietnam veterans who have post-traumatic stress disorder often develop the same disorder themselves.

To investigate whether this phenomenon occurred among social workers who offered their services during the September 11, 2001 attacks, Boscarino and his colleagues mailed questionnaires in May 2003, to 600 social workers who had addresses in New York City.

Overall, 236 social workers returned the questionnaires. More than 80 percent said they counseled people during the days following the attacks.

The investigators found that the more social workers had involved themselves in the recovery from the attacks, the more likely they were to have developed secondary trauma. However, the more social workers rated their work environment as being supportive, the less likely they were to develop secondary trauma.

These findings, reported in the International Journal of Emergency Mental Health, reinforce the importance of creating a good work environment for people exposed to traumatized patients on a regular basis, Boscarino noted.

He added that although the September 11 attacks were a unique event, social workers, psychologists and psychiatrists who regularly counsel abused women, for instance, may also be at risk of secondary trauma.

"This could be an occupational hazard that needs to be looked at," he said.

SOURCE: *International Journal of Emergency Mental Health, June 2004.*

Reuters, July 1, 2004.

It is believed that those who have experienced prior traumatic events may be at a higher risk to develop PTSD from a new event, while those for whom this is the first exposure to a traumatic event may have more emotional resilience to handle it. Some even suggest that there are different genetic vulnerabilities in response to stress and trauma. Studies have shown that people who have a more positive outlook on life—that is, those who believe that "a glass is half full rather than half empty"— may have more resilience in handling trauma. Some people learn to shut off their painful emotions so they may not feel emotional pain during a crisis or trauma situation. Others may have developed a very distinct coping style that permits them to go on. In this last group there may be those who escaped from terrorism in their native country. However, there are some theories that suggest a loss of resilience each time another trauma event is experienced.

The one most important factor found, however, in studies that looked at survival techniques was the presence of a support system made up of caring people. The more support a person perceived he or she had, the less emotional impact from the current trauma, no matter what kind of trauma it was. This is also true for crisis intervention when a non-traumatic but emotionally distressing crisis occurs. Although emotionally painful when experiencing them, crisis periods can be considered positive for personal growth afterwards. For example, the death of a parent may be a very painful event when it occurs, but the sense of relief that a loved one is no longer suffering and the ability to reclaim one's own life can be very positive outcomes for those who were caretakers. We more fully describe the techniques recommended in dealing with crisis and trauma in Chapter Ten.

Seriously Mentally Ill

What about the police officer who responds to a call at an apartment house and discovers that the door is locked? He or she knocks loudly and calls out for someone. Nothing is heard at first. Then slowly the door opens slightly with the woman inside peering out. There is enough space for the officer to slam open the door, but that could traumatize the family. The right choice is to stand or sit there talking quietly to the person to avoid getting him or her more upset. Once the person seems calmer, it may be possible to persuade him or her to open the door and leave peacefully. Police officers trained in dealing with the mentally ill or in hostage negotiation techniques have far fewer deaths or serious injuries because of their ability to "talk down" someone who is suffering from severe mental illness.

Some mentally ill people become aggressive when confronted with a legal situation. Many police departments are beginning to carry laser guns to protect themselves when responding to a crisis call with someone they know has been diagnosed as mentally ill. Look at this description of the taser in Box 1.2 and imagine what it feels like getting stunned by it.

Adults who are seriously mentally ill may react inappropriately to a fire fighter or emergency medical technician who has come to help them. If the person is responding to his or her own internal mental stimuli, the mentally ill adult may be confused by the identity of the First Responder and may respond in a disorganized or even aggressive manner. This behavior is likely when severely mentally ill persons stop taking their anti-psychotic medication and are out of touch with reality. As with Stacey who described in Box 1.3, the risk for the First Responder

BOX 1.2

Taser Guns Growing in Popularity

Firing 50,000 volts of electricity into a person's body is an extreme measure, but at least it's better than a bullet. That may be the ultimate lesson to draw from the experiences of police departments that have issued to their officers.

The number of people killed by police in Seattle, Miami, Phoenix, and other cities has fallen dramatically, in part, it seems, because officers in those cities have been relying on Taser guns when, in the past, they might have used deadly force.

But as the Taser spreads rapidly, it is raising questions about whether the weapon, which can also be applied directly to the skin as a stun gun, could be abused by the police. The Taser zaps suspects with 50,000 volts of electricity, disabling them for five seconds at a time. Critics say the weapon is ripe for abuse because the shock leaves no obvious mark, other than what looks like a small bee sting. Human rights groups in the United States and abroad have called Tasers potential instruments of torture.

Incidents of abuse are not unknown. A man in Las Vegas died last month after being shot with a Taser four or five times. Here's what his cousin saw:

"He was on the ground," Ms. Bell said in a telephone interview. "He had two pairs of handcuffs on him, and I didn't know the Taser was being used until I heard him screaming. He kept screaming and screaming, saying, 'Oh God, Jesus, please no.' He was screaming in pain, he was hurt and he didn't resist."

The long term effects of being zapped with 50,000 volts are unknown, and the possible lethality of the weapon is open to debate. Still, if the alternative is the use of a gun that will almost certainly cause serious injury or death, police departments should seriously consider training officers in the use of a Taser.

Police departments should vigilantly guard against the abusive use of Taser guns, just as they should guard against abuse of any kind. Policies limiting the use of Taser guns should be strictly enforced, so that officers are held accountable if they resort to a Taser gun when safer and less painful methods can safely be used to obtain an offender's compliance.

by TChris

Posted Sunday: March 07, 2004

Taser Guns

---

is to exacerbate the situation by setting off a violent attack by the person who otherwise would not be aggressive. It is important for the First Responder to learn how to recognize the difference between a mentally ill or substance abusing person and one who is purposefully dangerous or behaving aggressively.

We describe the major mental illnesses and the role of First Responders in dealing with them in Chapters Five (psychotic behavior), Six (mood disorders), and Seven (anxiety disorders), in addition to the personality disorders in Chapter Eight and the substance use disorders in Chapter Nine.

Children

Children who have mental problems pose a difficult problem for First Responders. Those children with limited intellectual resources may be easily tricked into giving a statement if the interviewer asks questions that can be answered by yes or no. The problems associated with mental

---

BOX 1.3

Stacey

Stacey had recently moved to a new city with her mother after experiencing a violent rape when three boys who were much bigger than she attacked her. She made some new friends with kids her age (16) and accepted their invitation to hang out with them one Saturday evening. Unbeknownst to her, there was a curfew for 16 year olds and younger. The police came to where she and her friends were just hanging out and hassled them. Stacey had her money and new lipstick in a special zippered compartment in her backpack.

A group of about ten teens were in the parking lot of a restaurant when the police car drove up. Some of the teens scattered but Stacey and one other boy didn't move. Stacey says later she felt like she was paralyzed, like a "deer in headlights" when the police stopped the car and a man and a woman police officer got out. The female officer grabbed Stacey's backpack and rifled through it, perhaps looking for identification. Her $20 bill and new lipstick fell to the pavement. She asked the officer to please put her money and lipstick back in the bag.

The officer ignored Stacey's pleas and left the lipstick and money on the floor. She said something that Stacey felt was nasty and started walking closer to Stacey.

"Don't touch me." Stacey screamed frantically again and again as the officer approached her. Her cries grew louder and she began fighting off the officer as soon as she began patting down Stacey. Fortunately, others in the parking lot saw and heard the interchange and started yelling so that the officer finally stopped touching her.

However, Stacey was arrested, handcuffed and taken down to the station house. When her mother came down to get her, she informed the police about Stacey's rape and her fears about being touched by someone she didn't know.

Could the officer have approached Stacey in a different way to have avoided the arrest and subsequent legal charges?

---

retardation are chronic and they will not go away with a quick fix. Those who have emotional problems also need special handling by the First Responder. In the above case (see Box 1.3), a girl who had been raped one year earlier and then was stopped by the police for being out after curfew, could have had a different ending had the first responder here been more sensitive to her mental condition at the time.

Was Stacey just behaving like a typical teenager when she wanted her money and lipstick preserved? Could the police officer have known that Stacey had recently been raped and had such a reaction to being touched as a result? No, but she could have known that this was one possible reason for Stacey's frantic behavior as the officer approached her. We discuss various ways to approach teens and avoid exacerbating trauma reactions that had left scars previously, as well techniques to deal with those teens with serious mental disorders in Chapter Twelve.

A child protective worker was called to the house by a neighbor who feared that a child was being harmed. Box 1.4 describes the situation that a CPS worker found when she entered Linda's home. It became clear rapidly that Linda had a serious mental illness. It took longer to recognize that there was no baby to protect.

Other cases involve police officers who are about to make an arrest. It is important here to interact with mentally disturbed individuals, both children and adults, in a way that does not exacerbate their

---

BOX 1.4

Linda

Linda was sitting in her home sobbing and wringing her hands when Denise, the CPS worker assigned to her case rang the bell. A neighbor had called in the complaint stating that Linda's baby was missing.

The neighbor had rung Linda's bell and when Linda answered the door sobbing, the neighbor learned that Linda was upset because she couldn't find her baby.

When the CPS worker got to the home, Linda was sitting fairly motionless.

The CPS worker asked question after question but couldn't get any information from Linda. She was so new to town that she had no friends or support system.

After awhile, the picture became clearer. Linda did not have a baby anymore. Rather, her children were grown and living on their own. Linda, who had been diagnosed with schizoaffective disorder, was mourning the fact that her daughter was now an adult and no longer a baby.

The missing baby was really a delusion.

Can Linda pose as a danger to the health and safety of the CPS worker?

---

illnesses. Law enforcement officers in various jurisdictions are getting training in making decisions about the mentally ill based on assessing and observing behavior, emotions, false beliefs, appearance, speech and thinking. They are trained to quickly identify hallucinations, delusions, suicidal and homicidal thoughts and behavior. Police officers who attend these programs around the country find them very helpful in their work.

DEPARTMENT OF JUSTICE, THE MILITARY AND THE MENTALLY ILL

The U.S. Department of Justice has become aware of the burgeoning numbers of mentally ill who are in the justice system. Jails and prisons estimate that close to 60% of their inmates have mental health problems. Close to 50% may have serious alcohol and other drug addictions that need attention to prevent recidivism. These numbers are substantially higher for women detainees and prisoners. We discuss the new therapeutic or problem-solving courts such as mental health courts, drug courts and domestic violence courts where restorative justice is the norm in Chapter Eleven. In Box 1.5 the interview with Judge Ginger Lerner-Wren, who sits on a misdemeanor mental health court in Broward County, Florida describes the community needs that accompany a mental health court.

Those old enough to remember stories about World War II and Viet Nam may remember that some men who did not want to go into combat preferred the socially stigmatizing label of 4F which meant they had mental problems and, therefore, were ineligible for the draft. In fact, many of the standardized psychological tests whose updated versions we use today were first developed during the 1950s to screen out the mentally ill or provide better services for them when they returned

BOX 1.5

Excerpts from a Conversation with the Judge of the First Mental Health Court

Face to Face: A Conversation with Judge Ginger Lerner-Wren

The judge discusses the stigma and reality of mental illness.

Q: Judge Lerner-Wren, it's no secret that the recidivism rate for the mentally ill in the criminal justice system is very high. What should be done about that?

A: Well, first of all, the recidivism rate as it relates to those individuals, for example, going through Broward's mental health court is not very high. We actually have a recidivism rate that, I think, floats at about 12%, which is extremely wonderful. Which means that when individuals who need mental health care get access to it and there is a mechanism for ensuring that the care is sufficient and continuous, people respond extremely well to treatment and live very wonderfully in the community.

Q: Are the county's mental health courts working as well as they should?

A: I don't think that these courts were ever supposed to be a panacea. I don't think that the issue that often gets focused on, in terms of the criminalization of the mentally ill, should be *the* primary focus of any policymaker or journalist. I think that the symptom of the criminalization of the mentally ill is a shameful, shameful trend. But the underlying causes of that, I really think, should be the focus, and that has to do with the high fragmentation of services in communities, the rationing of care, the lack of access to health insurance that covers mental health care, and just the overall stigma that surrounds these disorders and this illness generally.

Q: You've spoken of the need to "build capacity for treatment" in this community. What do you mean by that?

A: That means that communities have a full array of treatment and services for children and for adults that really spans the lifespan. It includes traditional psychiatric treatment, medications, psychotherapy, counseling, substance abuse treatment, but it also includes more than that.

It includes services and supports like housing, like access to disability benefits, case management services, day treatment services, and that's really what we're talking about.

The theory is, if we have communities that could really adequately provide the care to individuals with mental health needs, then you would not have people constantly recycling through jails and hospitals and the streets. We'd be able to meet their needs better.

Q: Do you think the community can afford that kind of full array of treatment over the lifespan of an individual, considering that there are many such individuals?

A: I do. I think that our governmental leadership, our policymakers, have not really been wise about the cost-effectiveness of providing care. The consequences of *not* having well-developed mental health care systems have been enormous, both in wastes, as far as over-utilization of hospitals and jails, to loss of productivity for employers.... Absenteeism is a huge issue in this country. The president commissioned data [that] supports economic loss, for example, just from productivity, in the millions. And so the waste of *not*— from a policy standpoint—treating mental health issues as we do other medical care issues has been enormous.

Q: Some people have proposed building a forensic hospital to treat the mentally ill once they enter the criminal justice system. Would such a hospital be helpful?

A: I wouldn't advocate for that. I think that we know what we need, in terms of different types of programs and housing. I think that if individuals can be safely and appropriately in the community, they can be and they should be. Where there are individuals that need forensic hospitalizations, which really is a very nice word for a jail, we have sufficient jail space in the county. And so, monies really need to go into the community, where they belong.

Q: In 2003, the President's New Freedom Commission on Mental Health, of which you were a member, recommended "a fundamental transformation of the nation's approach to mental health care." Yet little seems to have changed. Why is that?

A: I think a lot has changed, but it hasn't trickled down across the states yet. But on the federal level, there's been a tremendous amount of change, through the Department of Health and Human Services. The agency for substance use and mental health has gone through their own implementation process nationally, meaning that they're working on the national level to bring all of these federal agencies into alignment, consistent with the recommendations, and also reaching out to the states, to advocacy groups, to practitioners, policymakers, to educate about the recommendations of the president's commission report. And so I think that we're starting to see change happen, but transformation is clearly not an overnight process. Different states are implementing in their own way.

Q: Are the county and state spending enough on mental health care, and if not, how much should they be spending?

A: No. 1, they're not spending enough, and they have historically *not* spent enough, because for some reason these mental health issues have not been given the kind of prioritization that they really deserve. I'm not sure that the policymakers in our state understand that we are not going to be able to build and develop a strong workforce, for example, if we don't have healthy families and children that could succeed in school. And all of these issues are directly related to good mental health. And so there's got to be an investment—a strong, clear investment—in our mental health care delivery system in this state in order for us to really have a very strong citizenry.

Q: Why is there such a problem of access to mental health care? Is it just that there are too many patients and not enough providers, or is there more to it than that?

A: There's a little more to it than that. It's a combination of a lack of enough, just a lack of treatment and services generally, services and treatment systems that we have [are] highly, highly fragmented, not well organized, very, very difficult to get information, know who to call. If a parent wants help for their child, the schools don't have enough counselors, they don't

necessarily address the issues from a therapeutic way. For example, if a child behaves poorly in school, they may not see that as a mental health issue, they may see that as a behavioral problem and not make any recommendations, for example, for evaluation.

One thing we learned from the President's Commission is that the earlier one intervenes for mental health, the better. And one of the recommendations clearly is that all children should be evaluated on mental health issues, and evaluated early, in whatever setting, whether it be the pediatrician's office or a school-based clinic or some other fashion. Early intervention leads to prevention.

Q: What's the best way to educate the public about the problems of the mentally ill?

A: I think the best way is really through very, very strong educational and anti-stigma campaigns. You know, one in five individuals have some kind of mental health disorder. It's not just this mythical, stereotypic idea or image of, you know, a scary homeless person muttering on a street. It's our mothers, it's our fathers, it's our grandparents, it's our children. It's individuals who suffer from severe depression and they're too ashamed to talk about it. The research shows only half of individuals that suffer from depression ever seek care. We have to recognize that mental health issues are just the same as having any other kind of physical or medical condition, and that requires treatment, and there's absolutely no shame in going to see a doctor, for example, if you have a cardiac condition, and I think that's the education that we need to keep promoting: that these are real, authentic medical conditions, and we have to become much more enlightened about that.

Q: Is there anything else you'd like to say?

A: I just really want to emphasize that treatment works, treatment works for individuals with some of the most profoundly disabling conditions ... that we are all human beings, and that if there are medical conditions that require treatment, jails should never be used as an alternative to hospitals or health care.

BOX 1.5 (Continued)

Q: What if a mentally ill person commits a crime?

A: You know, again, I think that if a mentally ill person commits a crime, and there's public safety issues at stake, and it's a really serious offense, and no alternative to incarceration, for example, is appropriate, then that's why we have forensic hospitals. But the criminalization of the mentally ill has really not been about that. It's been about using jails as alternative hospitals. And so, to lose sight of the tragedy and the shame of that, I think, would be a mistake.

Interviewed by Editorial Writer Timothy Dodson

Background

Judge Ginger Lerner-Wren was elected a county court judge for the 17th judicial circuit in 1996. In 1997, she was selected to preside over the nation's first mental health court, dedicated to the decriminalization and treatment of the mentally ill in the criminal justice system.

Hailed as a national model, Broward County's mental health court was profiled at the White House Conference on Mental Health in 1999.

In July 2002, President Bush appointed Lerner-Wren to the President's New Freedom Commission on Mental Health, where she headed the Criminal Justice Subcommittee.

She currently serves on the National Advisory Council for the Substance Abuse and Mental Health Services Administration, continuing efforts to see that the presidential commission's recommendations are implemented nationwide.

Copyright © January 30, 2005, South Florida Sun-Sentinel

from war. Today, in the all volunteer military in the United States of America, there are mentally ill men and women who join, as well as those who are exposed to trauma and become mentally ill while in the military. Women and men returning from Desert Storm, Afghanistan, and now Iraq tell of terrible skin rashes and trouble breathing, along with high levels of anxiety disorders, including PTSD, mood disorders, and even psychotic breakdowns. The Veterans Administration Hospitals routinely care for these mentally ill former soldiers while the base clinics and specialty hospitals provide needed services for those still on active duty. Although we think of PTSD in connection with combat, it appears that many of the other mental illnesses are also commonplace, and they are treated in the mental health units on the bases, both in the United States and at temporary sites in combat zones. Those who serve as military police and emergency medical technicians in these military hospitals need to know what to expect when they encounter someone with a severe mental illness as well.

SUGGESTED READINGS

Brodsky, S. L. (2004). *Coping with cross examination and other pathways to effective testimony*. Washington, DC: American Psychological Association.

Constanza, M. (2004). *Psychology applied to law*. Belmont, CA: Wadsworth.

Fagan, T. J. & Ax, R. K. (Eds.). (2003). *Correctional mental health handbook*. Thousand Oaks, CA: Sage.

Schwartz, B. K. (2003). *Correctional psychology: Practice, programming, & administration*. Kingston, NJ: Civic Research Institute.

Walker, L. E. A. & Shapiro, D. L. (2004). *Introduction to forensic psychology: Clinical and social psychology perspectives*. New York: Kluwer/Plenum/Springer.

Wrightsman, L. S. (2001). *Forensic psychology*. Belmont, CA: Wadsworth.

Wrightsman, L. S., Greene, E., Nietzel, M. T., & Fortune, W. H. (2002). *Psychology and the legal system* (5th ed.). Belmont, CA: Wadsworth.

CHAPTER 2

Normal vs. Abnormal Behavior: A Continuum

A common question posed to every mental health expert by the "person on the street" is "Who is really normal?" The answer to the question is very complex and one that is open to significant areas of disagreement among professionals. To understand the issue more clearly, let us first consider the concept of normality and abnormality in the area of physical health and disease.

When someone is feeling ill and manifesting symptoms of pain, muscle aches, coughing and dizziness, the physician will take his or her temperature, look into his or her throat and ears and typically take blood and a swab of the patient's throat for analysis. When the physician discovers that the temperature is 102° F, the throat is red, the throat culture reveals bacteria and the person's blood values are askew, the diagnostician can safely say the patient is "abnormal." These "signs" of illness are objective, easily verifiable and would generally be agreed upon as abnormal by all experts. When we apply this "medical" or "disease" model of abnormality to psychological and psychiatric illness, however, agreement over what behaviors represent abnormality is not so clear cut.

In deciding whether psychological symptoms and behavior are "sick" or abnormal, mental health professionals do not typically rely on objective, physical evidence like blood tests, X-rays, or CAT scans. The decision to diagnose an individual as psychiatrically ill or abnormal is far more subjective and relies on clinical judgments that are influenced to some extent by a number of factors that take into consideration the appropriateness of people's behavior in the context of their environment, the effect of their behavior on others, and their culture as well as that of the judge making the evaluation of normality vs. abnormality. While each of these factors is important, no single one can be used to definitively label a person's behavior as "abnormal." We will discuss some of these factors in this chapter.

The Diagnostic and Statistical Manual of the American Psychiatric Association lists symptoms and behaviors for a variety of disorders to enable professionals to "diagnose" a patient and thus view him or her as "abnormal." Each of these disorders typically involves several symptoms that must be present in order for the diagnosis to be made. However, no single symptom or behavior can be assumed unequivocally to equal abnormality. Some individuals may feel that anxiety is "abnormal," yet it is quite normal when we face dangerous situations. The desire and intent to kill another human being may be seen as a sign of abnormality until we remember that we award medals to soldiers for killing our enemy. Self-mutilation sounds clearly sick until we recognize that tattoos and piercings are common today. The point is that these behaviors and symptoms, when viewed alone, do not provide the basis for an "abnormal" label. We must take the social context and the culture into account as well. This is not usually the case in medical abnormalities. A virus is a virus regardless of the context.

We also rely on statistics as a yardstick to define normality and abnormality. What is statistically most frequent or common in the population may be considered "normal" and what is infrequent or occurs less often would be labeled "abnormal." While we often use this model to assist us in evaluating behavior, especially in psychological testing, it has serious flaws. Most importantly, common or normal reactions may be considered abnormal at times. Many people, civilian and military, participated in the Holocaust that involved nearly annihilating an entire race of people. Despite the numbers of people involved, it would not be realistic to view their behavior as normal. Yet when many of Hitler's top lieutenants were formally evaluated psychologically, their actual responses were quite average or "normal" in a purely psychological sense. In summary, what is common in a population is not necessarily normal in the context in which we are attempting to understand it and cannot stand alone in defining these terms. There is no question that the ability to conform or behave like most people is useful in coping with and adjusting to the demands of life, but it is not usually an end in and of itself.

Often, the general population views abnormality in very simplistic terms that lead them to label others as sick in a very circular manner. For instance, some assume without question that if an individual has ever been labeled with a psychiatric diagnosis, then he or she is by definition "abnormal." They never ask who labeled that person or on what basis the label was assigned. In effect, abnormality becomes what the professional says it is, regardless of the basis of that judgment. Another potential error occurs when someone is seen as abnormal when he or she has been admitted to a psychiatric hospital. While that certainly should be a strong indication of psychiatric illness, community and cultural standards and values are often involved with that decision. Obnoxious teenagers, delinquents, and children whose parents become frustrated with them can often find themselves hospitalized for reasons that do not really reflect true psychological abnormality. Many subcultures within our society tolerate the idiosyncrasies of their members and never would consider them "abnormal" or admit them to a hospital. Move them out of that subculture, and they may immediately find themselves viewed as mentally ill.

Psychologist David Rosenhan and his colleagues performed a classic study in the early 1970s in which he sent eight of his graduate students into psychiatric admissions offices to act as pseudo patients. They were told only to complain of hearing a voice say "thud" or "empty." Every pseudo patient was admitted to an inpatient unit, but after admission, feigned no other symptoms or strange behavior. They behaved normally and made no further attempt to present as sick. Nevertheless, the staff continued to view them as ill, interpreting all of their behavior from the prism of the original diagnosis of psychosis. If they walked around the ward when they were bored, staff interpreted that behavior as resulting from anxiety. If they became appropriately angry at an attendant who mistreated them, they were seen as projecting the rage stemming from some delusion. In effect, every normal behavior was viewed as abnormal. When the pseudo patients were finally discharged after an average of 19 days, all were diagnosed as Schizophrenia, Residual Type. Here we see a most vivid example of the power of a psychiatric diagnosis and how even trained staff perceive abnormality in the most subjective way, based solely a single and ultimately faked symptom ("thud.").

As a result of the rather subjective nature of psychiatric diagnosis and the ambiguity surrounding the concept of abnormality, many researchers and clinicians have challenged the application of the medical or disease model to psychological problems. Albert Bandura, a noted psychologist, has written that psychopathology or "abnormality" is really a function of social judgments we make when others deviate from social norms regarding "appropriate" behavior. He describes this as social labeling of deviant behavior. He goes on to list several bases we use in making these social judgments.

First, we take into consideration the appropriateness of the individuals' behavior to a particular situation. If we experience the consequences of their behavior as positive, we view the behavior as positive. If it has a negative effect on us, their behavior now is labeled as deviant. A very quiet police recruit who rarely speaks and never challenges a very rigid, demanding sergeant may be seen as extremely cooperative and pleasant. When the same recruit goes to a SWAT team simulation and is expected by the training officer to be active and aggressive, his identical behavior may be seen as depressed and uncooperative. The behavior did not change, but the evaluation of its appropriateness to the situation had.

A second basis of social judgment revolves around behavioral deficits or the lack of necessary skills and behaviors to cope with problems. These deficits are labeled as symptoms of disorders when consequences are troublesome and problems are handled poorly. A firefighter who is promoted to Assistant Chief may have difficulty disciplining his men because he is concerned that they "like" him. He has great difficulty in setting limits, ordering others to perform tasks and may be labeled by his superiors as "needy," "dependent," and "insecure." When he is demoted to a basic firefighter position, the same behavior is perceived as "cooperative" and "non-authoritarian." The only thing that has changed is the role he played. In one role he is labeled "deviant" and in the other as quite healthy.

The ability of the judge to understand the actor's intention is a third basis of social judgment. When an individual's intention or motivation for a particular act is not understood, that behavior is likely to be labeled as deviant or mentally ill. Take the example of a teenage boy who follows an elderly woman into an alley noticing that she has a very big purse. He walks up to her, strikes her on the head with a crowbar and leaves the scene without taking anything. How would a police officer typically label that behavior, as a sign of delinquency or as a product of psychiatric illness? Imagine the same scenario, but this time the boy takes the purse. Delinquency or mental illness? When the intention for striking her does not appear obvious and is not understood by the officer, the most typical perception is that the behavior would be labeled mental illness, while the more obvious, "understandable" behavior that involved stealing would be seen as delinquency. Remember that the assaultive behavior is identical in both situations. Basically, when we do not understand someone's behavior, we are prone to call it mental illness. How does the judgment of the assaultive behavior change if we suggest that in the first example, the teenager was required to assault the woman as part of his induction into a street gang?

The personal attributes of an individual like age, sex, and occupation serve as a fourth basis of judgment. Certain behaviors are considered appropriate for one sex or at one age, but not for others. One gender-based example involves assertiveness. Assertive men in leadership roles often are considered strong, "go-getting," and competent, while women displaying the same behavior are frequently labeled as aggressive, mean spirited, and controlling. Thumb sucking at two years old is perceived as quite normal, until the very same behavior manifests itself at ten years old when it is viewed quite negatively as a sign of emotional problems. In these examples, the behavior is labeled "abnormal" as a function of a personal characteristic rather than on the nature of the behavior itself.

Keep in mind that the value and social judgments that come into play in these examples of behavior play a far more insignificant role in the diagnosis of physical illness. Consequently, it is incumbent on us to be aware of our own values, background and culture when we evaluate an individual's behavior as "abnormal."

As we can see, our ability to define abnormality and normality is a highly complex process involving a number of factors. Regardless of the complexity, First Responders will be called upon regularly to make these judgments and will need some basic criteria to support their decisions. The following represent fairly broad areas that define abnormality in rather abstract terms. More specific information regarding several psychiatric disorders and how to recognize them will be provided in the subsequent chapters.

Defective psychological functioning is one major criterion of abnormality. Specifically, impairments in attention, concentration, perception, judgment and memory all result in serious behavioral problems, including disorders like dementia, attention deficit disorder, psychosis and depression. When these functions are disturbed, judgments of abnormality are typically made. Defective social functioning is a second criterion of psychopathology. Here we will encounter mentally ill individuals who cannot refrain from engaging in behavior that is drastically at variance with the cultural norm. This is in contrast to the criminal who is more typically unwilling, rather than unable, to conform. Signs in our culture of defective social functioning include inadequate control of aggression, significant distrust and suspicion, and the inability for self-care and autonomy. A related criterion is basic loss of control. Many individuals are unable to control not only aggression, but their thoughts, fears and moods. Obsessive-compulsive patients are plagued by unwanted thoughts and rituals; phobic individuals understand intellectually that a bridge is safe to cross, but cannot bring themselves to drive over it; bipolar patients are tormented by their mood swings which seem to have a life of their own. They are all out of control. Society, including law enforcement officers, firefighters and emergency medical personnel, also serve to define abnormality along with family friends and mental health professionals. As we saw above, we all make social judgments that play an important role in how others are viewed. Finally, the last criterion of abnormality is the self-evaluation of our own behavior and feelings. Feelings of anxiety, depression, guilt and general subjective distress will play a very significant role in understanding abnormality and represent the most common basis for an individual to seek help from mental health professionals.

SUGGESTED READINGS

Bandura, A. (1969). *Principles of behavior modification*. New York: Holt, Rinehart and Winston.

Broman, C. L. (1996). Coping with personal problems. In H. W. Neighbors & J. S. Jackson (Eds.), *Mental health in black America* (pp. 117–129). Thousand Oaks, CA: Sage.

Cooper, C. R. & Denner, J. (1998). Theories linking culture and psychopathology: Universal and community-specific processes. *Annual review of psychology, 49*, 559–584.

Druss, B. G., Marcus, S. C., Rosenheck, R. A., Olfson, M., Tanielian, T., & Pincus, H. A. (2000). Understanding disability in mental and general medical conditions. *American Journal of Psychiatry, 157*, 1485–1491.

Elliott, C. (1996). *The rules of insanity: Moral responsibility and the mentally ill offender*. Albany: SUNY Press.

Humber, J. M., & Almeder, R. F. (Eds.). (1997). *What is Disease?* Totowa, NJ: Humana Press.

Rosenhan, D. L. (1973). On being sane in insane places, *Science, 179*, 250–258.

Strack, S. (Ed.). (2006). *Differentiating normal and abnormal personality*. New York: Springer Publishing Company.

Szasz, T. (1961). *The myth of mental illness: Foundations of a theory of personal conduct*. New York: Hoeber-Harper.

U.S. Department of Health and Human Services. (1999). *Mental health: A report of the Surgeon General*. Rockville, MD: Author.

Wakefield, J. C. (1992). The concept of mental disorder: On the boundary between biological facts and social values. *American psychologist 47* (3), 373–388, 371–472.

CHAPTER 3

Key Mental Health Issues in the Criminal Justice and Emergency Medical Systems

INTRODUCTION

The first two chapters in this book have attempted to describe how complex it is to define a mental illness as opposed to a simple physical illness. It is common knowledge that if people cough and sneeze, their throats hurt, and they have a slight fever, they may have a cold, allergy or other similar disease. Many of the *signs* (what can be observed) and *symptoms* (what is experienced) that accompany mental illnesses overlap and make them more complicated to diagnose. Some of these signs and symptoms, albeit at a milder level, are with us from time to time. For example, most of us have felt anxious, sad or depressed at times. Some students reading this book who expect to take an examination afterwards may feel some anxiety as they read and study, especially if there are new terms that must be learned. If others watched as that student studied, they might notice signs such as a tic, hand wringing, the twist of a piece of paper, a rash or other physical indication of anxiety. Those persons might also feel symptoms of nervousness, upset stomach, or headache, but unless they disclosed these feelings to others, they might not be known. Most people are more forgetful and inattentive, and they cannot concentrate as well when something is bothering them. They may even have a sleepless night or two. Children may wake up with nightmares or night terrors from time to time, but that doesn't give them a mental illness. However, it is not only the kinds and patterns of signs and symptoms that people experience, but also the strength and the length of time or pervasiveness of those symptoms that help us make a diagnosis.

It is important for all health service providers such as doctors, physician assistants, nurses, emergency medical technicians, psychologists, social workers, mental health counselors and others who work in the health industry to have an organized way to speak about signs and symptoms so that treatment interventions can be formulated. Those who interact with them, such as law enforcement officers and other first responders, must learn what signs and symptoms are important in making diagnoses and treatment planning so that the health providers have access to their accurate information from as close to the beginning as possible. This is part of what is called a *seamless health delivery service*, and it maximizes the possibility of the person's recovery. The basic way of communicating signs and symptoms that impact a person's health is to use one of two systems of categorization or *nosologies*. However, it is important to remember that the same signs and symptoms may be reflective of someone's culture, gender, or experience and are not indicative of a mental illness. This caution is found at the beginning of all nosology systems to make sure that they are not misused either inadvertently or for political or some other purpose.

DIAGNOSTIC CLASSIFICATION SYSTEMS

The World Health Organization (WHO), understanding that most health providers believe that the mind and body affect each other, classifies mental and physical diseases in the *International Classification of Diseases (ICD)*. Every 10 to 12 years this nosology is updated with new diseases or changes that have been found in disease patterns. It is published in most languages including English and is distributed around the world for health providers to use as a common language between them. Because it covers most known diseases, each section is necessarily brief. The American Psychiatric Association publishes a more comprehensive nosology of mental diseases and defects. This is called the *Diagnostic and Statistical Manual of Mental Disorders (DSM)*, and it is usually published during the same cycle as the ICD. At this time we are using the *ICD-10* and the *DSM-IV-TR*. The *DSM-IV-TR* actually was published midway in the cycle to permit the descriptions of the mental disorders to be updated, hence the addition of TR which stands for *Text Revisions*. The book has over 600 pages and criteria for over 300 different mental disorders listed; it also is published in different languages and used in many countries to collect statistics on the incidence and prevalence of different mental disorders. The major categories are outlined in Table 3.1.

The mental disorders that we will study in this book are those that are the most likely to impact the people with whom First Responders will have major contact. They can be divided into seven major groups as shown in Table 3.1. The different groups demonstrate variations in *cognition* or the way we think, *affect* or the way we feel, and *behavior* or the way we act. The latter part of this chapter will discuss the various ways to measure patterns of thinking, emotions, and actions through observations, clinical interviews and psychological tests and the types of typical interventions within the criminal justice and medical systems. But first, let's look at the different groups.

Table 3.1. Diagnosis Covered in this Text

A. Organic Brain Syndromes or Cognitive Disorders
   a. Delirium
   b. Dementias
   c. Amnesic Disorders
   d. Seizure Disorders
   e. Mental Retardation & Developmental Disorders

B. Psychotic Disorders
   a. Schizophrenias
   b. Delusional Disorder
   c. Brief Psychotic Disorder
   d. Schizoaffective Disorder

C. Mood Disorders
   a. Major Depressive Disorder (MDD)
     i. Major Depressive Episode
     ii. Dysthymic Disorder
   b. BiPolar Disorder
     i. Bipolar I
     ii. Bipolar II
     iii. Cyclothymic Disorder

D. Anxiety Disorders
   a. Panic Disorder
   b. General Anxiety Disorder (GAD)
   c. Phobic Disorder
   d. Separation Anxiety Disorder
   e. Obsessive Compulsive Disorder (OCD)
   f. Post Traumatic Stress Disorder (PTSD)

E. Somatoform Disorders
   a. Hypochondriasis
   b. Conversion Disorders
   c. Pain Disorders
   d. Body Dysmorphic Disorder

F. Dissociative Disorders
   a. Dissociative Amnesia
   b. Dissociative Fugue
   c. Dissociative Identity Disorder (formerly Multiple Personality Disorder)

G. Personality Disorders
   a. Schizoid Personality Disorder
   b. Schizotypal Personality Disorder
   c. Paranoid Personality Disorder
   d. Avoidant Personality Disorder
   e. Dependent Personality Disorder
   f. Obsessive Compulsive Personality Disorder
   g. Histrionic Personality Disorder
   h. Narcissistic Personality Disorder
   i. Borderline Personality Disorder
   j. Anti-Social Personality Disorder
     i. Psychopath

(Continued)

Table 3.1. (Continued)

H. Substance Abuse Disorders
  a. Depressants
    i. Alcohol
    ii. Sedative, hypnotic & anxiolytic substances
  b. Stimulants
    i. Amphetamines & methamphetamines
    ii. Cocaine & crack
  c. Opioids
    i. Heroin
  d. Hallucinogens
    i. Marijuana
    ii. LSD
  e. Other Abused Drugs
    i. PCP, Ecstasy, Ketamine, GBH
    ii. Steroids
    iii. Inhalants

MAJOR DIAGNOSTIC CATEGORIES

Organic Brain Disorders and Cognitive Disorders

Organic Brain Disorders currently described in *DSM-IV-TR* as *Cognitive Disorders* have a major impact on brain functions that control the entire nervous system. These disorders affect voluntary and involuntary movements of the body, such as in Parkinson's or seizure disorders, as well as cognitive functions including memory, judgment and the ability to think manifested in dementia and mental retardation. The next chapter describes each of the major Cognitive Disorders and how the nervous system works in more detail. It is important to note that these disorders usually mean that a part of the nervous system has been damaged or destroyed, either by disease or defect (usually from genetics, birth or subsequent injury), and this damage can have a major impact on the entire body and mind. Scientists have found that cells in the nervous system cannot regenerate, although new studies suggest that some nerve cells can replicate themselves naturally, while others may be able to do so with some additional help, such as introduction of new genetic material from *stem* cells that are in embryonic and undifferentiated forms. The damage from disorders such as *cerebral vascular incident* or *stroke* is stable but irreversible, while that from the *dementias* or *Multiple Sclerosis* continues to increase despite our best efforts. Sometimes healthy nerve cells can be trained to take over the functions of the damaged cells through *biofeedback* and other types of interventions. Other times the best intervention is to protect the safety and comfort of the person. New proposed research using stem cells is described in Box 3.1.

Many of the signs and symptoms of Cognitive Disorders are also found in other disorders in which there is no demonstrable damage or

BOX 3.1

Congressional Committee Hearing Covers Embryonic Stem Cell Research Scandal

By Steven Ertelt
LifeNews.com Editor
March 8, 2006

Washington, DC (LifeNews.com)—A Congressional committee held hearings on the fallout from the international embryonic stem cell research scandal in South Korea where a team of scientists falsified research supposedly showing the controversial science making significant progress.

Lawmakers debated the ethical problems surrounding the research, including the need to destroy human embryos and obtaining donations of human eggs for research.

Rep. Mark Souder, Republican chairman of the subcommittee said he was disturbed by reports that women in South Korea were paid by scientists for their eggs—which could result in coercion or taking advantage of poor women.

Souder told the scientists and bureaucrats who attended the hearing not to treat members of Congress "like little children" by minimizing the ramifications of the scandal.

"This scientific scandal is not an isolated incident of fabrication, without real application to US research efforts," he said.

"Rather, it highlights the serious, inherent potential problems with research cloning and embryonic stem cell research, including but not limited to: exploitation, fraud, and coercion."

Meanwhile, Richard Doerflinger, the deputy director of Pro-Life Activities at the U.S. Conference of Catholic Bishops and a bioethics watchdog, told the committee that there are scientific, political and moral lessons to be learned about the South Korea scandal.

Doerflinger explained that the scientific lesson is not to trust claims that human cloning has been successful, pointing to false claims in years past.

Politically, Doerflinger said human cloning and embryonic stem cell research shouldn't get a free pass—especially since the research has yet to make any progress in curing or helping people.

"The political agenda for cloning has long been divorced from the facts," he said, according to a Catholic Online report.

"To win public support and government funding, advocates for human cloning and ESC (embryonic stem cell) research have long made hyped claims and exaggerated promises to legislators and the public," Doerflinger explained.

Advocates of embryonic stem cell research chided pro-life lawmakers, with Rep. Elijah Cummings, a Maryland Democrat, saying "opponents of embryonic stem cell research seem to have difficulty containing their glee" at the South Korean scandal.

He and Democratic Rep. Henry Waxman of California said that it would be wrong to limit the unproven research despite the problems. They said new ethics guidelines should be adopted instead.

The House of Representatives Government Reform subcommittee on criminal justice and drug policy held the hearing.

Among those called as witnesses were directors of the NIH Stem Cell Task Force, the National Institute on Deafness and Other Communication Disorders, the Office for Human Research Protections, the Office of Research Integrity, and several professors of life sciences.

Printed from: http://www.lifenews.com/ bio1370.html

defect in the brain. However, this is not to suggest that there are no underlying neurochemical dysfunctions in the brain that are responsible for emotions and behavior. It may be possible to reverse or change the functioning of the person with these disorders through psychotherapy, medication, changing the situation or other interventions. Therefore, it is important to separate out the cognitive, organically based disorders from these other disorders. A good assessment including detailed descriptions of observations of the person's behavior will help in the proper diagnosis.

In the past, non-organically based disorders were divided into two categories—*psychotic* or out of touch with reality and *neurotic*—or emotionally crippling. Today, more accurate descriptors are used that divide what used to be called "neurotic" into *Mood Disorders* involving alterations in affective regulation; *Somatoform* disorders that involve symptoms that mimic real physical illness; *Anxiety* disorders that are primarily characterized by an excessive degree of anxious feelings; and *Dissociative* disorders involving alterations in consciousness. None of these disorders result from any measurable impairment to the brain or central nervous system. Understanding the impact of these disorders on a person may assist the First Responder in the best methods of relating to people who are afflicted with them.

Psychotic Disorders

Psychotic disorders, including *Schizophrenia, Delusional Disorder, Brief Psychotic Disorder and Schizoaffective Disorder* are those that render people's emotions and cognitive processes dysfunctional and their reality testing impaired. If people live in a fantasy world, respond to internal stimuli such as hallucinations and delusions, and are not able to control their emotions, they may be suffering from a psychotic disorder. The most common ones are described in Chapter Five. It is important to remember that not everyone with a psychotic disorder is easy to diagnose, especially since many of the symptoms are internal to the person, are not always present, and must be reported to the evaluator. Since there is often secondary gain for someone with many symptoms of a psychotic disorder in the criminal justice system, it is important to assess for malingering in these cases. For others, the stigma and shame still associated with serious mental illness may make them less likely to report their symptoms.

Mood Disorders

Mood Disorders are those that impair people's ability to regulate their emotions. Major mood disorders include *Major Depressive Disorder, Dysthymia, BiPolar Disorder and Cyclothymia.* Depression, the common cold of mental illness, involves periods of sadness and hopelessness. Sometimes mood cycles back and forth from depression to a high energy, excited and expansive state in which the person may be extremely active, pleasure oriented, and euphoric, often engaging in inappropriate behavior. This is called BiPolar Disorder. As is discussed in Chapter Six, BiPolar Disorder, especially the type that rapidly cycles between high and low moods, is very difficult to treat.

Anxiety, Somatoform and Dissociative Disorders

Anxiety, Somatoform and Dissociative Disorders, as well as some of the Mood Disorders discussed above, are believed to be caused, in part, by a person's biological and genetic makeup, in part by psychological conditioning, and in part by environmental or social conditions. Since most behavior occurs on a continuum ranging from minimal to maximum display, it is important to understand what is motivating or propelling a specific observable behavioral sign. The culture in which someone has been raised plays an important part in the baseline on the behavioral continuum. Recent studies in basic sciences, such as neuroanatomy and neurophysiology, chemistry, and pharmakinetics, have provided important information about the circuitry of the brain and its neurochemical transmitters. For example, it is now known that disorders impacting on thinking, that is, cognition, are mediated by too much or too little of certain neurochemicals that are needed for optimum functioning of the nervous system, while those disorders that affect the emotions are mediated by other neurochemical circuitry.

Anxiety Disorders cause people to feel uneasy and fearful because the anxiety often is globally experienced rather than associated with a specific object or situation. *General Anxiety Disorder* or GAD involves chronic worry over many areas and chronic muscle tension. *Panic Disorder* involves bodily symptoms that are regulated by the autonomic nervous system. Here people often cannot breathe, experience heart palpitations, and feel as if they are about to die from a heart attack. Paramedics and law enforcement can be trained to tell the difference between those who are experiencing a coronary from those who are having a genuine panic attack. *Post Traumatic Stress Disorder* (PTSD) is considered an anxiety disorder because of the prominence of the hyperarousal of the body and nervous system.

Somatoform Disorders may reflect anxiety in an indirect way. One type of Somatoform Disorder is *Conversion Disorder* in which psychological conflict is unconsciously converted into bodily symptoms in the form of sensory or motor impairments. For example, a person engaged in a heated argument with his or her partner suddenly develops a paralyzed arm that does not follow the physiological pathway of the nerves or muscles and has absolutely no physical basis. A more recent example is the case of Cambodian women refugees who developed an idiopathic blindness even though their eyes were physically intact.

Dissociative Disorders are represented by disorders that involve alterations in consciousness and significant memory loss with no physical basis. The most notable and most frequently portrayed in books and movies is *Dissociative Identity Disorders* or Multiple Personality Disorder.

Personality and Substance Use Disorders

Personality Disorders are often questioned by some as if they are not truly mental disorders. These disorders are the most troubling in the *DSM-IV-TR* in terms of reliability and validity. Most people with a personality disorder manifest traits that result in interpersonal difficulties for themselves and others. Although the *DSM-IV-TR* lists different types of personality disorders, these categories are the least reliable and most controversial of all the diagnoses. Personality Disorders, however, represent an important category for people who get in trouble with the law and therefore will be discussed in Chapter Eight.

Substance Use Disorders are among the most prevalent psychiatric disorders and will be covered in Chapter Nine. These disorders are often *co-morbid* or co-occurring with other psychiatric illness and always represent a major challenge for First Responders

CLINICAL ASSESSMENT

Clinical assessment of whether a person has a mental disorder or not is a complex process that includes collecting different observations and measurements of behavior in a variety of ways. A clinical assessment is usually conducted in order to make a specific *diagnosis* of a mental disorder, so, it is important to follow a systematic method in order to compare one individual to others who have been found to have the same diagnosis. Generally, this systematic method must use *reliable* and *valid* measurement techniques so a comprehensive evaluation of the person's biological, psychological and social factors will result. *Reliability* means that different mental health workers would come to the same diagnosis using the same criteria no matter where they were trained or where they might live. *Validity* means that the criteria used actually do measure what they are supposed to measure.

Most people have experience in using their observational skills to look at someone carefully and compare that person's total functioning with what is known about human behavior. To do this, we need to know something about developmental psychology or what we would expect from someone who is the same age, level of intellectual abilities and judgment, racial and cultural background, ability to manage emotions, and social functioning. Although it may not be done formally, a number of hypotheses or ideas are created in the clinician's mind about how this person functions in each of the areas that must be measured and then the data are integrated while drawing comparisons from the appropriate group. Often general answers to the hypotheses are developed, such as "this person is functioning like a 2-year old" if the person is having a temper tantrum or "she is dressing like a teenager" if someone is wearing a t-shirt and ripped jeans. If more precision in this process is needed, psychological tests that are standardized for measuring samples of behavior of people of different ages and characteristics can be used. Then the individual can be compared to the group on which that test was standardized. All these factors are pulled together, weighed in terms of relevance, and then a diagnosis is formulated. Often the diagnostic criteria for several different mental disorders must be compared with other information before we are satisfied with the diagnosis or diagnoses selected. This is called making a *differential diagnosis*, and it can become quite complex when the person's signs and symptoms cut across more than one diagnostic category.

Standards for Assessment Technique Development

Assessment techniques are subjected to certain requirements to be sure that they measure what they are designed to measure. The major requirements are called *reliability, validity, and standardization*. There are scientific procedures to check on the reliability and validity of a test. Standardization of a psychological test is done using scientific methods so that one person's performance on that test can be compared to the group norms.

RELIABILITY. An assessment technique is considered reliable if anyone who uses it obtains consistent results. If a person presents the same group of signs and symptoms to ten different mental health clinicians, the assessment technique for those signs and symptoms would be considered reliable if all ten clinicians were able to come to the same diagnosis. Different clinicians may interpret the results differently, but if the results themselves are consistently obtained each time the technique is used, then the technique is considered reliable.

VALIDITY. An assessment technique is considered to be valid if it measures what it is purports to measure. There are different types of validity. For example, if a test for depression actually includes the signs and symptoms of depression, which is called *face* or *descriptive* validity. Using an established test as a way to see if a newer test will also measure depression is called *concurrent* validity. If a violence risk assessment technique is used to assess if the person will act out in a violent manner in the future, the technique is called *predictive validity*.

STANDARDIZATION. Many assessments use a procedure to make sure that their instrument is consistent (reliable) and measures what it is designed to measure (valid) using statistical methods. This process is called standardization, and it creates a set of norms against which an individual can be measured. Psychologists like to use standardized tests in addition to observational data and clinical interviews in order to make a diagnosis.

Standardized tests used to assess different areas are called a *standardized test battery*, and the process usually includes observations, clinical interviews and mental status examination, together with standardized cognitive and personality tests. Additional tests to measure the impact from trauma may be used when the person has experienced an assault, domestic violence, sexual abuse, or other traumatic events. If there is a suspicion, history, or evidence of someone having committed a violent act, there may also be need to perform a violence or sexual offender risk assessment using special assessment inventories for this purpose.

Prior to the more careful development of reliable criteria with which to make a diagnosis, different mental health practitioners would differ on what certain signs and symptom meant.

Types of Assessment

OBSERVATION. It is important to develop objective observational skills in order to conduct a proper assessment for diagnosis or treatment planning. To do this, it is important to recount what is seen without putting an interpretation on the behavior. The behavior or actions are described in detail rather than attempting to explain or understand what the person is doing.

Behaviorists often use a simple observational rating scale to help organize what is observed. The A, B, C's of behavior can be recorded on a particular form. These are the Antecedents (or what happened before), the target Behavior itself, and the Consequences (or what will happen after such behavior occurred). Behaviorally oriented psychologists will help a person *operationally define* certain behaviors so that there can be greater reliability and validity in what behavior each person describes and labels. When a person looks for patterns in the observed behavior, then it may be called *self-monitoring* or *self-observation*. There are a number of formal checklists and behavior rating scales that are published to assess behavior in particular settings or areas. Some simply count whether a behavior occurred or not during specific time periods while others rate the frequency or strength of a behavior on a 5-point or 7-point rating scale.

CLINICAL INTERVIEW. The clinical interview usually consists of a series of questions and answers that occurs between the interviewer and interviewee. It is an important way to obtain information about the problem that brought the person into the clinician's office, called the *presenting problem*, as well as to obtain relevant histories from the interviewee. The traditional clinical interview is usually a series of open-ended questions with the interviewer conducting further follow-up questions in relevant areas, or it can be more structured, with the questions prepared prior to the interview. This is called a *structured interview* and may be preferred when it is important not to forget to ask for information across a number of different areas. The structured interview also is preferred when there is a time limit on the interview because it gets to the essential questions quickly. Many believe that the open-ended clinical interview allows for more rapport and trust to be established for it gives the individual more time to think about answers to the questions asked. There are many different published assessment forms for various types of structured and semi-structured interviews.

MENTAL STATUS EXAMINATION. Behavioral observations that are made in a systematic way during the clinical interview, called a *mental status exam*, assess mental state in a general way, to see if a mental disorder is present and, if so, what type of disorder it might be. Five specific areas are typically assessed during a *mental status exam* listed in Table 3.2. These are *appearance and behavior, thought processes and content, mood and affect, cognitive functioning*, and *judgment and insight*. To assess for appearance and behavior, the person's overt behavior, clothing, posture, expressions, cleanliness and general appearance are observed. Thought processes can be measured by listening to how the person talks, what vocabulary words are used, is the speech coherent and organized, how rapid or slow is it, how loud or soft is the tone, and is there any evidence of hallucinations or delusions as will be described in later chapters on dementias and psychotic thoughts.

The third area in the mental status exam is *mood* and *affect*. Affect is defined as an observed emotional state at a particular time while mood is a more pervasive, internal emotional state that often lasts a longer period of time and characterizes the general feeling state of the person. Evidence of what we call a flat or blunted mood, sadness, depression, high levels of activity and manic states are assessed. It is important to match the person's mood with his or her behavior. For example, is the person describing a happy event but appears as if he or she is about to cry? It is important how pervasive is the affect that is presented. Is the affect based on a particular event or does it seem more likely to be the predominant mood?

Table 3.2. Steps in a Mental Status Exam

1. Appearance and behavior
2. Thought processes
3. Mood and affect
4. Intellectual functioning
5. Senses

The fourth area to be assessed in a mental status exam is the person's intellectual and cognitive functioning. Here it is important to determine if the person's vocabulary level is the same as his or her educational level. Look for evidence that the person's knowledge is inconsistent with educational background, possibly due to a neuropsychological or emotional deficit. Does it appear that the person had a higher capacity to function at an earlier time and has now regressed, or is he or she just as able to function today as he or she did at an earlier time? Does the person have a good awareness of his or her surroundings? Does the person know the time, where they are, as well as who the evaluator or she or he is? If the answer is yes, then the person is said to be *oriented in all spheres.*

Finally, the patient's *insight and judgment* are evaluated to determine their appreciation of their problems and their ability to exercise good judgment in solving common problems.

Standardized Psychological Tests

COGNITIVE TESTS. The two major cognitive areas measured by standardized psychological tests are intelligence and neuropsychological functioning. The standardized intelligence test used by most psychologists is the *Weschler Adult Intelligence Scale-Third Edition (WAIS-III).* This test yields three IQ scores, one for verbal areas, one for performance areas, and a total or Full Scale IQ. It also yields information about the person's memory and the number of resources available for cognitive problem solving. In addition to gaining an understanding of the person's intellectual functioning as compared to the standardized norms for his or her age, each area thought to be important in cognitive functioning such as social comprehension and skills, abstract thinking and reasoning, ability to analyze and synthesize concepts, attention to details, short- and long-term memory, and perceptual organization is assessed and compared to norms both for the individual's other abilities and with others on whom the test was standardized. It is also possible to determine what, if any, cognitive skills might be impacted by an emotional disorder by analyzing the individual subtests in the test battery.

The *Weschler Intelligence Scale for Children-Fourth Edition (WISC-IV)* and the *WPSSI* are used for children and preschool children respectively. A shortened form of the WAIS called the *Weschler Abbreviated Scale of Intelligence (WASI)* can be used to obtain a good estimate of intellectual ability when there is not enough time to administer the entire WAIS. There are numerous other tests of cognitive functioning that can be used both in schools and in other agencies, such as the *Stanford-Binet, Peabody Picture Vocabulary Test,* but the Weschler tests are the most widely used in the field.

Neuropsychological tests can measure specific cognitive functions and deficits in the various areas of the brain and nervous system that may be first noticed in behavior or other screening instruments. The

Weschler Memory Scales-Third Edition (WMS-III) is often used together with the WAIS to assess for more details in memory functioning, which is often negatively impacted in someone who has brain dysfunction. The *Repeatable Battery for the Assessment of Neurological Symptoms (RBANS)* is another screening instrument to give further information about areas that might be negatively impacting on cognitive functioning. The two major neurological assessment batteries that are used by neuropsychologists to measure a variety of areas in more depth are the *Halstead-Reitan* and the *Luria-Nebraska*. Each one has a series of sub-tests, and an individual's performance is compared to the standardized norms developed for each area.

Although these tests are all widely used by psychologists and neuropsychologists, it is important to remember that brain function is difficult to measure because what is normal may vary widely amongst people in a heterogeneous population. If the individual who is being evaluated is from a population that was not included in the standardization sample, then the norms will not apply to him or her. Thus, if those who do not speak English as their first language need to take the test, they should be compared to others from their own cultural group for reliable and valid results. It is also important to remember that if a test is not administered in the exact way that the instructions dictate, then the norms may not be appropriate to use for comparisons. This can literally cost someone their life if the IQ points fall above or below a certain cut off score such as when considering whether someone has the requisite mental state to be executed. Read about the dilemma discussed in Virginia's Daryl Atkins' case in Box 3.2.

In addition to neuropsychological tests, people with cognitive deficits should have a complete physical examination with neuroimaging of the structure and function of the brain. Some of the newer computerized neurological diagnostic tests are further discussed in the next chapter. Integration of the findings from physical, psychological, and environmental assessment can best provide the information upon which to base a diagnosis involving cognitive deficits.

PERSONALITY TESTS. There are two major types of personality tests that are used today in a standardized psychological test battery. *Objective personality inventories* such as the *Minnesota Multiphasic Personality Inventory (MMPI-2)* or the *Personality Assessment Inventory (PAI)* are simple to administer and score and usually have a computerized profile of the results available. *Projective Tests* such as the *Rorschach* and the *Thematic Apperception Test* (TAT) are more subjective to administer, score, and interpret and, therefore, may be less reliable than a self-administered inventory.

The MMPI-2 and the adolescent version, MMPI-A are widely used in the forensic setting because they are the oldest and they set the standard for comparing one person's scored profile against the group on which the test was standardized. In fact, the test, which was first published over

BOX 3.2

Inmate's Rising I.Q. Score Could Mean his Death
By Adam Liptak—NY Times

YORKTOWN, Va., Feb. 3—Three years ago, in the case of a Virginia man named Daryl R. Atkins, the United States Supreme Court ruled that it was unconstitutional to execute the mentally retarded. But Mr. Atkins's recent test scores could eliminate him from that group.

His scores have shot up, a defense expert said, thanks to the mental workout his participation in years of litigation gave him.

The Supreme Court, which did not decide whether Mr. Atkins was retarded, noted that he scored 59 on an I.Q. test in 1998. The cutoff for retardation in Virginia is 70.

A defense expert who retested Mr. Atkins last year found that his I.Q. was 74. In court here on Thursday, prosecutors said their expert's latest test yielded 76.

Mr. Atkins, a slight, balding 27-year-old in an orange jumpsuit, sat slumped with his chin on his hand as lawyers argued about whether his intelligence was low enough to spare him from execution. In 1996, he and another man abducted Eric Nesbitt, 21, an airman from Langley Air Force Base, forced him to withdraw money from an A.T.M. and then shot him eight times, killing him.

He will be one of the first death row inmates to have a jury trial on the question of whether he is retarded. The jury's decision will determine whether his life will be spared.

Mr. Atkins's more recent scores should be discounted, a clinical psychologist who tested him in 1998 and 2004 said, because they are the result of "a forced march towards increased mental stimulation" provided by the case itself.

"Oddly enough, because of his constant contact with the many lawyers that worked on his case," the psychologist, Dr. Evan S. Nelson, wrote in a report in November, "Mr. Atkins received more intellectual stimulation in prison than he did during his late adolescence and early adulthood. That included practicing his reading and writing skills, learning about abstract legal concepts and communicating with professionals."

In helping put an end to the death penalty for the mentally retarded, then, Mr. Atkins could have ensured his own execution.

Prosecutors say that Mr. Atkins has never been retarded and that the recent tests confirm it. "I don't see how a 76 is exculpatory and evidence of mental retardation," Eileen M. Addison, the commonwealth's attorney here, said in court on Thursday. "It needs to be under 70."

Ms. Addison has said that Mr. Atkins's crime also proves that he is not retarded. In an interview last year, she said that his ability to load and work a gun, to recognize an A.T.M. card, to direct Mr. Nesbitt to withdraw money and to identify a remote area for the killing all proved that Mr. Atkins is not retarded.

"I don't believe the truly mentally retarded commit these kinds of crimes," she said last year. She did not respond to recent messages seeking comment.

There are several other reasons that Mr. Atkins's scores may have risen. I.Q. scores are rarely completely stable and can drift, though within a relatively narrow range, typically by five points up or down. Psychologists recognize that practice drives scores higher. And I.Q.'s tend to rise over time, by about three points a decade.

Dr. Evans, the defense psychologist, concluded that "Mr. Atkins's 'true' I.Q. is somewhere in the mid- to upper 60s."

60 years ago, was restandardized over 20 years ago making interpretation more relevant to today's culture and norms. The test itself contains 567 true or false statements that the person can answer on a separate answer sheet that then gets fed into the computer by the examiner or sent to the company for scoring. The computerized version has available an interpretative report which some clinicians like because it offers an acceptable

Dozens of mentally retarded people have been released from death row as a consequence of the Supreme Court's decision, under agreements and judicial findings. Others will face trials like Mr. Atkins's. David M. Gossett, a Washington lawyer who represents a death row inmate in a similar position in Georgia, said incarceration itself may also have a positive effect on the test scores.

"Prisons are highly structured and safe environments," Mr. Gossett said. "They're sometimes good environments for the mentally retarded. These people are not vegetables. They can learn. These are people who can get better at taking tests."

In old cases and new ones, courts across the country have been struggling to interpret the Supreme Court's decision. Seven states have passed new laws, according to the Death Penalty Information Center.

They have adopted essentially the same definition of mental retardation, requiring defendants to prove three things: that their I.Q. is below 70 or 75, that they lack fundamental social and practical skills, and that both conditions existed before they turned 18.

Mr. Atkins was never tested as a youth, and so the jury will have to consider how to look back using his test scores as a young adult.

The defense bears the burden of proving he is retarded, so the absence of scores from when he was young and the relatively high current test numbers may hurt his case.

"I don't know what you have before age 18," Judge Prentis Smiley Jr., of the York County Circuit Court here, told Mr. Atkins's lawyers on Thursday. "That's your problem."

The judge described a clear standard. "The issues are bright lights and targeted with a bull's-eye," Judge Smiley said.

Richard Burr, who represents Mr. Atkins along with Joseph A. Migliozzi Jr., disagreed.

"For people real close to the edge, there is nothing easy about that," Mr. Burr said. "There is going to be controverted evidence, subject to sharp disputes and disagreements."

Jurors in Mr. Atkins's case, which will be tried this spring or summer, will probably hear from mental health experts, teachers, family members, classmates and, perhaps, victims of some of the 16 other felonies that Mr. Atkins committed when he was 18 in what Dr. Nelson called a four-month crime spree. He dropped out of high school that year, his third attempt to pass the tenth grade.

Virginia's handling of mental retardation in capital cases is relatively unusual. In new cases, juries in this state do not reach the question until after they have convicted the defendant. Many other states have a judge decide the issue before trial.

Judge Smiley said he planned to tell jurors that Mr. Atkins was convicted and sentenced to death. He will also allow prosecutors to dismiss jurors who say they oppose the death penalty in all circumstances.

Mr. Atkins's lawyers asked the Virginia Supreme Court to reverse those rulings. On Wednesday, that court declined to hear the case.

"This proceeding has veered off the course of fairness," Mr. Burr told Judge Smiley on Thursday. "We want to have the opportunity to prove that Daryl Atkins is mentally retarded."

Mr. Atkins nodded in agreement.

NY Times
February 6, 2005

interpretation of what the profiles mean. However, the interpretations can be misused without taking into account the social and cultural history of the client and conditions under which the test is administered. It can also be hand scored, although this is very time consuming and fraught with opportunities to make mistakes. There are several validity scales that can help determine if test-takers have made a valid test-taking effort or if their answers indicate their responses were influenced by their feeling very bad or very good at the time they take the test.

The PAI has an administration and scoring system similar to those of the MMPI. However, the test-takers' choose from four different responses rather than the true/false responses on the MMPI. The computerized profiles are normed on both a clinical and non-clinical population that yields less pathology than does the MMPI. It also has better scales to assess for Post Traumatic Stress Disorders. Other simple inventories to administer to assess for specific disorders include the *Beck Anxiety Inventory (BAI)* and *Beck Depression Inventory (BDI)*, and Speilberger's *State-Trait Anger Inventory (STAXI)*. While there are many other standardized tests that assist in the assessment of emotional disorders, these are the most common ones used in forensic settings.

The *Rorschach Ink Blot* test was developed over 80 years ago by a Swiss psychoanalyst, Hermann Rorschach. It is designed to understand how a person organizes a series of ambiguous and unstructured stimuli that are inkblots. There are ten black inkblots on white cards, in addition to some also having color as part of the design. The examiner hands one card at a time to the person who is asked to tell what he or she sees in it. The method is based on the belief that someone's personality can be inferred from the way he or she organizes perceptions and projects them onto what he or she sees in the cards. There are several different scoring systems available for the Rorschach although it remained controversial until the *Comprehensive System* was developed using research by Exner. The Exner system, as it is often called, requires a standardized way to administer the cards and score the perceptions, which then can be entered into the computer, and all the computations and interpretations are received on a printout. Although still not perfect and not accepted by all psychologists, the Exner system has helped standardize a complex but useful assessment technique. It is especially useful with bright clients who may be defensive on the inventories but more willing to be creative with the inkblots.

The same criticisms about the Rorschach have also been leveled against the TAT, also popularized about 80 years ago. This test consists of 31 cards of pictures, some actual famous art hanging in museums. The instructions suggest choosing ten cards and asking the examinee to make up a story with a beginning, middle and end to it. The themes that are seen in the various stories are analyzed together with the results of the clinical interview and other tests that might have been administered. Since there are no reliability or validity norms for the TAT, it cannot be considered a standardized test, but many clinicians use it along with other tests as an important source of a different kind of behavioral information.

TRAUMA TESTS. Assessment of the impact from trauma events has gained in popularity in the last 10 years with the development of standardized tests to assist in that measurement. The most popular test is the *Traumatic Symptom Inventory* (TSI) that is based on the research of John Briere, PhD. The test lists a series of signs and symptoms typically seen in those who have experienced a traumatic event and normed on subjects from physical and sexual assault centers. Results are given in a graph format that is interpreted similarly to the MMPI tests. A newer test, also based on Briere's research, is the *Detailed Assessment of Posttraumatic Stress (DAPS)*. It utilizes signs and symptoms from a person's life and determines if they produced emotional reactions strong enough to cause a PTSD disorder. Edna Foa, PhD, also a psychologist, developed a different standardized test to measure PTSD symptoms, from her research. Dissociation, a component often seen in those who have developed PTSD, can be assessed using several different inventories. Fears can be measured using the *Modified Fear Survey (MFS)* first developed by Wolpe and later adapted for sexual assault victims by Kilpatrick.

VIOLENCE RISK ASSESSMENT. A 20-year study by the MacArthur Foundation has helped in better understanding of the assessment of the risk of violence by developing a core list of risk factors using actuarial methodology. See examples in Table 3.3.

Actuarial assessments such as the *Violence Risk Assessment Guide (VRAG), Sex Offender Risk Assessment Guide (SORAG), Minnesota Sex Offender Screening Tool (MSOST), Historical Clinical Risk-20 (HCR-20)*, and the *Hare Psychopathy Check List-Revised (PCL-R)*, and others are now being utilized by courts to help understand the risk of future violence, and to determine whether a particular individual should

Table 3.3. MacArthur Variables

- Demographic Variables
  - Age Range, Sex, SES
- Sociological Variables
  - Peers & family support violence
  - Economic Instability
  - Familiarity & skill with weapons
  - Size of potential victim pool
  - Particular pattern or random
- Biological Variables
  - History of head injury
  - Soft neurological signs
  - Abnormal neuropsychological findings
- Psychological Variables
  - Mental Disorders
  - Substance Abuse (most powerful predictor)
  - Poor Impulse Control
  - Low Intelligence

be released on probation, sentenced to outpatient treatment, or paroled. They are also being used to assist psychologists in recommending that predatory sex offenders be civilly committed after serving their prison sentences for sex crimes. Some organizational psychologists who are hired by businesses that want to lower their risk of workplace violence are using these actuarial factors in their hiring and promotion inventories. These are controversial, in part, because of their static nature that is based on unchangeable facts (e.g., "How old were you when you committed your first act of violence?" or "Were your parents married or separated when you grew up?" or "How long was your longest relationship?"). In addition, the standardization sample is usually from incarcerated offenders who are considered a small part of the general pool of offenders, yet these actuarial inventories are being used quite often with those who are from a different racial or ethnic culture group or other non-matching demographic group.

TESTS OF MALINGERING. In addition to the validity scales embedded in most of the standardized tests used to measure emotional disorders, there are several standardized tests that purport to measure whether someone is malingering or trying to fool the examiner into believing he or she has a mental illness for secondary gain such as not being held responsible for their otherwise criminal behavior. The two most common tests for malingering of emotional disorders are the *Structured Interview of Reported Symptoms* (SIRS) and the *Miller Forensic Assessment of Symptoms Test* (MFAST). Both of these tests have been standardized using comparative samples of people who are told to fake symptoms of a particular emotional disorder and those who have been diagnosed with such a disorder. In general, the number of symptoms selected as well as the pattern of symptoms help an examiner detect attempts to fake being mentally ill. There are also several tests that assist in the detection of faking neuropsychological symptoms, especially memory. These include the *Test of Memory Malingering* (TOMM) and the Frederick's *Validity Indicator Profile* (VIP).

A summary of the assessment instruments is listed in Box 3.3.

INTERVENTIONS. There are numerous interventions that mental health professionals can select from when trying to rehabilitate or remediate a mental disorder. The four most common ones used in the criminal justice system or by First Responders are psychopharmacology or medication, competency restoration, community-based psychotherapy, and hospitalization. As is discussed in Chapter Eleven, there is a world-wide effort, propelled by the human rights movement, to rehabilitate those people who commit crimes while mentally ill or adversely affected by substance abuse such as alcohol and other drugs. *Therapeutic* or *restorative justice*, as it is called, often includes decriminalizing the mentally ill and providing appropriate treatment in the community's mental health system which is monitored by the specialty courts. The following interventions, however, are more commonly found in the prisons and hospitals of the justice department.

PSYCHOPHARMACOLOGY OR MEDICATION. Most jails and prisons today give inmates who have mental health problems drugs to help keep them calm and manage them. Usually the generic form of medication is used as there are *formularies* or lists of approved drugs to keep the costs down. Nonetheless, the use of psychotropic drugs is still very costly, especially if it is carefully regulated with physical examinations and blood tests on a regularly scheduled basis and used in combination with psychotherapy. In selecting the drug or drugs that can be beneficial to the person, it is important to try different ones in the same class or even mix some together in what is sometimes called

BOX 3.4
Common Psychotropic Medications

Generic	Brand Name
MOOD DISORDERS	
MAO Inhibitors	
Deprenyl(Selegiline)	Selegiline or Eldepryl
Isocarboxazid	Marplan
Tranylcypromine	Parnate
Phenelzine	Nardil
Tricyclics	
Trimipramine	Surmontil
Desipramine	Norpramin
Doxepin	Sinequan
Amoxapine	Asendin
Maprotiline	Ludiomil
Protriptyline	Vivactil
Nortriptyline	Pamelor
Amitriptyline	Elavil
Imipramine	Tofranil
Clomipramine	Anafranil
SSRIs	
Citalopram	Celexa
Excitolopram	Lexapro
Fluvoxamine	Luvox
Paroxetine	Paxil
Sertraline	Zoloft
Fluoxetine	Prozac/Serafem
Other Antidepressants	
Trazodone	Desyrel
Nefazodone	Serzone

Generic	Brand Name
Buproprion	Wellbutrin SR/Zyban
Mirtazapine	Remeron
Venlafaxine	Effexor
Tetracyclic Compounds	
Amoxapine	Asendin
Maprotiline	Ludiomil
Mood Stabilizers	
Topiramate	Topamax
Gabapentin	Neurontin
Lamotrigine	Lamictal
Carbamazepine	Tegretol
Valproic Acid	Depakote
Tiagabine	Gabitril
PSYCHOTIC SYMPTOMS	
Traditional Anti-Psychotics	
Phenothiazines	
Chlorpromazine	Thorazine
Fluphenazine	Prolixin
Prochlorperazine	Compazine
Promethazine	
Thioridazine	Mellaril
Dibenzodiazepines	
Clozapine	Clozaril
Butyrphenomes	
Haloperidol	Haldol
Thioxanthenes	
Thiothixene	Navane

a *cocktail*. Obviously, this cannot be done when a limited formulary must be used. These drugs have powerful side effects and, if not properly regulated, can lead to other disorders, some of which may be permanent. For example, one of the most common permanent side effects is called *tardive dyskinesia*, which causes strange muscle movements such as thrusting the tongue in and out of the mouth or jerking of the arms and legs at irregular intervals. Newer drugs have fewer side effects, but they are usually not listed on the formularies because they are more expensive. The specific medications used for each mental condition will be further discussed in the following chapters, but a summary of the major classifications and chemical names is listed in Box 3.4.

Generic	Brand Name	Generic	Brand Name
Others		**ADD & ADHD**	
Trifluoperazine	Stelazine		
Pimozide	Orap		
Perphenazine	Trilafon	**Cognitive Enhancers**	
Molindone	Moban	Methylphenidate	Ritalin
Mesoridazine	Serentil	Pemoline	Cylert
Loxapine	Loxitane	Dextroamphetamine	
		and amphetamine	Adderall
Atypical Antipsychotics		Dextroamphetamine	
Ziprasidone	Geodon	sulfate	Dexedrine
Quetiapine	Seroquel	Modafinil	Provigil
Olanzapine	Zyprexa		Benzedrine
Risperidone	Risperdal	Clonidine	Catapres
Clozapine	Clozaril	Reboxetine	
Aripipresole	Abilify	Guanfacine	Tenex
		Bupropion	Wellbutrin
ANTI ANXIETY			
		DEMENTIA	
Benzodiazomines			
Anxiolytics		**Cognitive Enhancers**	
Alprazolam	Xanex	Donepezil	Arecept
Chlordoazepoxide	Librium	Rivastigmine	Exelon
Clonazepam	Klonopin	Galanthamine	Reminil
Chlorazepate	Tranxene		
Diazepam	Valium	PARKINSON'S DRUGS	
Lorazepam	Ativan		
Oxazepam	Serax	Pramipexole	Mirapex
Prazepam	Centrax	Ropinirole	Requip
		Tolcapone	
Other Anxiolytic Drugs		Entacapone	Sinemet
Buspirone	Buspar	Bromocriptine	
Hydroxyzine	Vistaril		
	Atarax		
Sleep Aids			
Zaleplon	Sonata		
Zolpidem	Ambien		

COMPETENCY RESTORATION. In most legal systems used today, a mentally ill person who commits an act that would be considered a crime if she or he had the requisite mental state, may not be found mentally competent to stand trial if certain conditions are met. These conditions are often referred to as the *Dusky standard* because the U.S. Supreme Court enumerated them in a case by that name [*Dusky v. U.S.*, USSC (1960)]. Most other countries have adopted similar standards as seen in Table 3.4 which include the ability to know what he or she is charged with, to know the role and function of a judge, defense and prosecuting attorneys, to know what are the different pleas and consequences of them should he or she be found guilty, and the ability to assist his or her attorney with *a reasonable degree of rational understanding.*

Table 3.4. Dusky Competency Criteria

1. Factual understanding of charges against him or her
2. Rational understanding of the legal procedure
   a. Role of prosecutor
   b. Role of defense attorney
   c. Role of judge
   d. Role of jury
   e. Different pleas available
   f. General appreciation of seriousness of charges
3. Reasonable ability to assist counsel
   a. Will the person's mental illness get in the way of helping Attorney to defend them
4. Is the person's mental health restorable?
5. If the person becomes competent, will he or she remain stable and competent

Notice how much emphasis there is on cognitive ability rather than on emotions or dysfunctional mood. In fact, unless a mood disorder, such as bipolar or depression, affects someone's ability to think and make judgments about these very specific issues, the person is considered competent to stand trial whether or not he or she is mentally ill.

Even with this strict definition of competency, many people who commit that which would otherwise be called a crime are found not competent to stand trial and are remanded to a hospital for treatment to restore their competency. In some cases, if the act was not one considered dangerous to themselves or others, they might be remanded to treatment in the community, but this is not a popular option if the person has committed other criminal acts in the past or is at high risk to commit another criminal act in the future.

PSYCHOTHERAPY. There are many different methods of psychotherapy today that are used to help the mentally ill ameliorate or reduce their bothersome symptoms or learn how to manage and cope with their illness. Different theories of the causation of the mental illness may dictate the type of psychotherapy utilized, and different mental health professionals are trained in a variety of these methodologies or strategies. Insight-oriented or dynamic psychotherapy, which may be based on psychoanalytic or humanistic theories, is often long term and has greater efficacy with people who are intelligent and are known to think about their psychological lives. It is not often used with those who have psychotic disorders unless hallucinations and delusions are controlled. Those who are considered seriously mentally ill may need a combination of medication, psychotherapy, and case management to help them live a symptom reduced or symptom free life. Psychotherapy in this case may be aimed at cognitive and behavioral aspects rather than attempts to regulate mood which may be controlled by the medication.

It is unusual to find psychotherapy available to those in jails or prisons. If it is provided, then it is more common to find psychotherapy that deals with cognitive-behavioral domains rather than insight-oriented psychotherapy since cognitive-behavioral techniques have been found to have efficacy with specific problems in a short-term dose. For example, cognitive-behavioral methods are often used in alcohol and drug rehabilitation programs in jails and prisons to teach people how to avoid using these substances to make themselves feel better. Specialty programs are also used in sex offender treatment units to try to prevent these defendants from committing the same offenses upon release. In some states there are procedures for civil commitment to special treatment programs for those who are adjudicated as sex predators. Cognitive-behavioral methods are also used for reducing anxiety and depression symptoms by teaching inmates how to regulate their emotions by changing their thought patterns.

There are some exceptions to a strict cognitive-behavioral approach that have been appearing in some newer programs that are still short-term and focused therapies. For example, some institutions have been using a form of EMDR (Eye Movement Desensitization Reintegration) therapy that has known efficacy with reducing the emotional impact from trauma. There has also been some experimentation with a modified version of Dialectical Behavior Therapy (DBT), a treatment known to have some efficacy with people who have been diagnosed with certain personality disorders.

Other types of therapy have been used in institutions, such as Reality Therapy which focuses on the connection between making poor judgments and emotions, and those therapies with different names that focus on changing or managing emotions and behavior. Women's prisons have found that therapies focusing on the stress of their family and social roles helpful, especially since so many of the women serving time have been abused at some point in their lives. Therapies that deal with dual diagnoses often include a combination of psychotherapy and drug treatment. One of the major difficulties has been finding a sufficient number of well-trained therapists to work in the prisons because so many of them are located in rural areas away from where most highly trained psychologists and psychiatrists live and work.

HOSPITALIZATION. Finally, as a last resort, those people who are mentally ill may have to spend some time in a psychiatric hospital. In some communities, there are sufficient numbers of the mentally ill to have a separate forensic hospital with locked facilities to protect the inmates and community. In most communities, there are hospitals for those who are committed in civil proceedings because they are found to be gravely mentally ill and a danger to themselves and/or others. There may be a forensic psychiatric unit in the state hospital where someone who is adjudicated incompetent to proceed to trial is transferred. If after a certain amount of time, usually 5 to 7 years, that person cannot be restored to competency but is still considered too dangerous to release into the community, the person may be transferred to the civil hospital. The average stay in these hospitals for someone who has not been involved with the criminal justice system is only a few months, so it is possible that there is a revolving door for those who are homeless and without family or other social support systems in the community to help them care for themselves.

In forensic hospitals or units, the average stay is approximately 18 months until they may be transferred to long-term facilities, especially for those who have been adjudicated *Not Guilty by Reason of Insanity* (NGRI). This decision is not only based on whether or not their mental illness has been "cured," but it is also dependent upon the crime they committed and their current level of dangerousness. While the general public believes that people who are found NGRI are somehow "getting away with being punished for their crime," in fact, studies have found that they are often locked up in the hospital for longer periods of time than those who are sent to prison for the same acts. In addition, it is the doctors and the courts who will determine what happens to them in the hospital, such as whether or not they are forced to take medication or enter into treatment programs, and when they are ready for release into the community, while in prison they have the right to self-determination as long as they are not behavior problems, and they have a definite time for their release unless they try to be paroled earlier.

SUGGESTED READINGS

American Psychiatric Association (2000). *Diagnostic & Statistical manual of mental disorders, text revision. (DSM-IV-TR)*. Washington, DC: American Psychiatric Press.

Beck, A. T. (1999). *Prisoners of hate: The cognitive basis of anger, hostility, & Violence*. New York: Harper/Collins.

Dorfman, W. I. & Hersen, M. (2001). *Understanding psychological assessment*. New York: Springer.

Olin, J. T. & Keatinge, C. (1998). *Rapid psychological assessment*. New York: Wiley.

Quinsey, V. L., Harris, G. T., Rice, M. E., & Cormier, C. A. (1998). *Violent offenders: Appraising and managing risk*. Washington, DC: American Psychological Association.

Shapiro, D. L. (1991). *Forensic psychological assessment: An integrative approach*. Boston: Allyn & Bacon.

Wettstein, R. M. (Ed.). (1998). *Treatment of offenders with mental disorders*. New York: Guilford.

Wolber, G. J. & Carne, W. F. (2002). *Writing psychological reports: A guide for clinicians. Second Edition*. Sarasota, FL: Professional Resources Press.

CHAPTER 4

Disorders of the Brain and Central Nervous System

Our brain and nervous system is the basic organ system that regulates our mental functions of thinking, feeling, and acting. We can divide the nervous system into two parts, the Central Nervous System (CNS) and the Peripheral Nervous System (PNS). The brain is located in the CNS while the neurons that deliver messages to and from the brain and the rest of the body are in the PNS. The PNS is divided into two major systems, the Somatic Nervous System that regulates our voluntary movements and the Autonomic Nervous System (ANS) that regulates our involuntary movements such as our emotions, breathing, heart rate, and blood pressure. The ANS is further divided into two sections, the sympathetic which expends energy and the parasympathetic which conserves energy. These systems all work together in a coordinated way, telling the body when to manufacture more or fewer neurochemicals called neurotransmitters that will facilitate or shut down the messages that go to and from the brain and make our body work.

Our thinking behavior is centralized in the cortex of the brain while our emotions are regulated in the other brain structures called the midbrain. Messages get carried up and down to various areas in the brain by bundles of nerve cells called neurons in the spinal cord and the rest of the body. These messages use chemicals and electric impulses to travel. Some neurons have a cover or sheath that covers it so that the electrical messages can travel faster. As you can imagine, a breakdown in the production, release, or elimination of some chemicals can cause a problem in the system. Damage to the nerve cells or the myelin sheaths that cover them can cause a problem with the system.

In this chapter, we have included diagrammatic pictures of how scientists believe these structures appear to help explain the structure and function of the various parts of the nervous system. We then go on to discuss some of the common disorders of the nervous system and brain that cause mental health problems. Throughout this book, we discuss mental health and mental illness as is commonly done using what is called an integrated approach. This means that the mind and the body function in an integrated way. Problems in the physical body may cause problems in the thinking, feeling, and behavioral areas controlled by the mind or the nervous system, and problems in the nervous system can cause physical difficulties. In psychology we call this the *biopsychosocial* approach. The BIO part is the role of the structure and functions in the brain and nervous system that are regulated by the DNA and other genetic components that we discuss more fully in this chapter. However, it is important to remember that biology is not always destiny, because in fact, the psychological state and the environment may potentiate or hinder most genetic biological factors.

Some scientists believe that all of our behavior can be understood through the biological and neuroscience mechanisms of the brain. Read through this chapter and then think about your position on this suggestion. Here are some pointers to help make a decision. Most of the signs and symptoms of mental illness that we discuss in this chapter and in the following ones can be explained by the neurochemistry. That is to say, if we do not have sufficient serotonin in the synapse, the nerve impulse may be slowed down and we feel depressed. Or, if we have too much dopamine there, we may not be able to think clearly as is true for those who are labeled with schizophrenia. We add a stimulant to those who have trouble with attention and concentration, use anti-anxiety medication for those who have panic attacks, and anti-depressants and mood stabilizers for those who have manic and depression swings. However, can we really measure what some call mindfulness or the internal workings of the mind by how many neurotransmitters are present in the synapse? Read on.

NERVE CELL

In Box 4.1 we have pictured a typical *nerve cell* that has a *cell body* where the *genetic material (DNA)* resides in a fluid called *cytoplasm*. The cell body has little projections on its ends called *dendrites*. These dendrites have little receptor cells that can both release and remove *neurotransmitters* from the space in between it and the next cell called the *synapse*. There is fluid in the synapse that contains various neurochemicals that change constantly. The other end of the nerve cell is called the *axon*. Axons are longer and also have projections on their ends called *end brushes*. These areas also have the ability to release chemicals or remove them from the space called the *synaptic cleft*. Nerve cells do not actually touch each other but, rather, the end brushes on the dendrites and those of the axon terminate in that space. The chemicals in the synapse help the message jump from one neuron to another. Bundles of nerve cells are called *neurons* and are found all over the body, although bundles of cell bodies are more likely to be found in the brain, and bundles of axons that connect to cell bodies in the brain can be found in the PNS throughout the body.

Box 4.1

Neuron

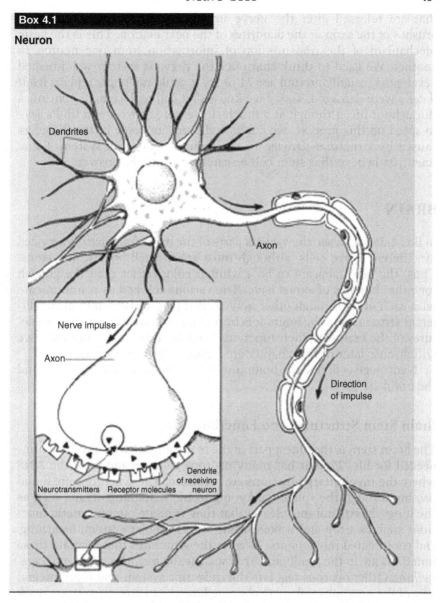

Most axons have nerve impulses that go one way-either to or from the brain. Axons are often very long structures, and they have nodules called *Nodes of Ranier* on regular intervals on their length that help speed the electrical impulses. When a nerve cell is stimulated, the message travels up or down it and then it rests. The nerve cells are stimulated by electrical impulses that are facilitated or slowed down by the neurochemical secretions that can be stored in little sacs before the synaptic cleft. These chemicals can be removed by other neurochemicals that are released after the nerve impulse passes, either in the end brushes of the axon or the dendrites of the next neuron. This is the basic mechanism of the transmission of information from one neuron to another. We used to think that once the nervous system was finished developing, usually around age 21 or so, it could no longer replace itself if cells were damaged. Today we know that cell replacement continues throughout life, although at a much slower rate. If we could find a way to speed up this process, we could find cures for some of the disorders caused by structural damage to the brain and nervous system. Some scientists believe that stem cell research will find the answer.

BRAIN

In Box 4.2 we can see the various parts of the brain. Each part is serviced by different nerve cells, although most are the cell bodies, not axons. Thus, the brain appears to be a whitish color rather than the grayish tone that bundles of axons have. The various cell bodies communicate with each other through other nerve cells that are also found in the different structures in the brain. It is important to know the different structures of the brain and their functions because many of the disorders we will discuss later in this chapter are regulated by these structures.

Neurologists divide the brain into two major parts: the *forebrain* and the *brain stem*.

Brain Stem Structures and Function

The brain stem is the oldest part of the brain and contains the structures needed for life. Thus it has many neurons going to and from the ANS where the involuntary functions are regulated. These neurons are found passing through the spinal cord going to life sustaining organs such as the lungs, heart, and muscles so that they regulate our automatic functions such as sleep and wakefulness, cardiovascular system, breathing, and coordinated movements. Most of the structures that regulate these functions are in the hindbrain areas such as the *medulla, pons, and cerebellum*. Other neurons regulate the endocrine system that is an integral part of the neurophysiology explaining how the neurotransmitters work as described below. *Hormones* are manufactured by the endocrine system, which are carried to the nervous system by the blood.

There are several other structures in the brain stem that are important to know because of their impact on our emotions. For example, the *reticular activating system*, (RAS) which regulates our arousal, tension and attention, is found in the midbrain area.

Above that but below the forebrain are the thalamus and hypothalamus which coordinate emotions and behavior. Some believe that they serve as a switching station because of their regulatory functions. The *limbic system*, which is just below the forebrain above the thalamus

BOX 4.2

Brain

Schematic side view (lateral) of the left hemisphere showing the frontal, temporal, parietal, and occipital lobes. The right hemisphere has the same lobes, sulci, and gyri. But the main language centers are lateralized to the left hemisphere. Broca's area controls speech production and Wernicke's area controls comprehension of language. The left hemisphere specializes in the brain's main language system, including expression and comprehension, speaking, writing, and reading. Damage to the posterior region of the left frontal lobe results in Broca's aphasia, a non-fluent type in which speech is hesitant, incomplete, and lacks syntax; damage in the posterior left superior temporal gyrus results in Wernicke's aphasia, a fluent aphasia in which speech is well articulated but does not make any sense and language comprehension is absent. Damage to other regions within the left hemisphere leads to other disturbances in language.

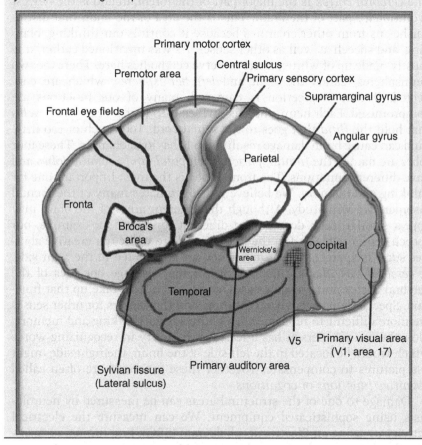

and hypothalamus, is implicated in many of the psychopathological conditions explained in the next chapters. It is made up of the *hippocampus, cingulated gyrus, septum, and amygdala*. This system helps regulate our emotional experiences and behavior involved in sex, aggression, hunger and thirst. It is also believed that the brain stem receives and stores emotional memories, particularly those that are associated with strong emotional experiences such as trauma. This may be why it is implicated in our ability to learn along with the cerebral cortex. To help those who develop PTSD after experiencing trauma control their memories, which are reexperienced as if the trauma were reoccurring when they remain in the midbrain area, it is important to transfer the memories into the cognitive memory area in the cerebral cortex as described below. The *basal ganglia* with the *caudate nucleus* are also located near the forebrain and control posture and motor activities.

Forebrain Structures and Function

The *cerebral cortex* is the major part of the forebrain and is the newest evolutionary part of the brain. This is the area of the brain that distinguishes us from other creatures because it controls our thinking, planning, and speech as well as other senses. As was mentioned earlier, it is mostly made up of white matter or nerve cell bodies here. There are two hemispheres, called the *right* and *left hemispheres*, which are connected. If that connection is damaged, many of our functions are compromised. Each hemisphere is divided into four lobes by *ventricles* that hold the *fluid* that goes to the spinal cord. Too much or too little fluid can cause brain damage resulting in behavioral changes. These four lobes are named the *frontal, parietal, temporal, and occipital lobes* and have different functions. The frontal lobe is the most important one for thinking and memory. We believe it also regulates many of the mental disorders we will study. Although the different areas of the brain may appear similar, each does have a different function. For example, our speech center is located in the left hemisphere while our creative abilities such as appreciation of music and art are located in the right side. A *cerebral vascular accident* or stroke may damage one area of the cerebral cortex and, in some cases, another area will take up that function. Speech, language, vision, hearing, and the centers for other senses are more difficult to replicate than pathways for thinking and memory. Nonetheless, if a person has a learning disability in recognizing words which would be located in the left side of the brain, the right side might use pictures to compensate. Together these functions are often called *cognitive functions* or *cognitions*.

Damage to one of the structural areas can be measured by neurologists using sophisticated equipment. We can measure the electrical activity by using an Electroencephalogram (EEG), find tumors or measure blood flow to the brain through a Magnetic Resonating Imaging machine (MRI), or other functions by Computerized Tomography (CT and PET scans). Damage to the various brain functions can be measured by neuropsychologists who know how a particular part of the brain should function on a particular task and how to use tests to measure the degree to which the function is working. Psychopharmacologists also can infer damage to the neurotransmitters by analyzing behavior that is known to be regulated by each chemical.

NEUROTRANSMITTERS

The function of neurotransmitters has only been recently studied by psychopharmacologists who are interested in manufacturing drugs that can better regulate the amount of a particular biochemical at the synapse. As has been previously mentioned, these researchers have found that the role of these biochemicals is to facilitate or slow down the nerve impulse transmission process. Thus, adding more of one or blocking the transmission of another may cure mental illnesses. There are several basic neurotransmitters that control the nerve impulses that jump from one neuron to another. Along with these neurotransmitters there are also other biochemicals that facilitate or slow down the nerve impulses. These are important to know as many of the behavioral changes we describe in later chapters are actually regulated by these neurotransmitters and therefore are implicated in the development of the particular symptoms of the mental illness. However, it is important to remember that the psychological and environmental conditions of the person are just as important in whether or not a change in the neurotransmitter will result in a mental illness, or if other bodily functions will release other biochemicals to compensate for the problem. In fact, the debate in the psychological community suggests that verbal psychotherapy is slower but just as efficient in producing changes in the neurotransmitters as taking the drugs, and there are fewer side effects.

The basic neurotransmitters that we will study are *serotonin, norepinephrine, dopamine, Gamma Aminobutric Acid (GABA), and Acetylcholine (ACh)*. But first we must learn a little about how they are regulated.

There are receptor cells in the nervous system that have an affinity to one or more of these neurotransmitters. Sometimes it is simply a question of which biochemical arrives at the receptor cell first, while, with others, they will only accept a particular biochemical. Some chemicals are *agonists* and facilitate the work of the neurotransmitter while others are *antagonists* and slow it down. Sometimes these biochemicals work together with enzymes and hormones to do their job. It is not necessary for our purposes to know all these different functions, but, rather, it is important to have a basic idea how they function in the nervous system.

The body has sensors in all the structures that manufacture some of these biochemicals which regulate when to produce more or less of it. When it learns it must produce more, this is called *up regulation*, and when it must make less, it is called *down regulation*. When a message comes down the path of a neuron, the biochemicals stored in vesicles at the end brushes are released into the synapse. Sometimes there is not enough of a particular neurotransmitter stored there, even though a sufficient supply is being manufactured. Other times, there may be too much of the neurotransmitter left in the synapse. After a message goes through the synapse to the next neuron, there are other biochemicals that cleanse the synapse from the neurotransmitters left there; this is called *reuptake*. If there is a problem in either case, some drugs will prevent the reuptake of those neurotransmitters so the next time a message comes through, an adequate supply of that biochemical is already in the synaptic cleft. The class of medications called Selective Serotonin Reuptake Inhibitors or SSRIs does this with serotonin which leaves a large enough supply of that neurotransmitter in the synapses and, thus, relieves some of the symptoms of depression or slower neuronal transmissions.

Serotonin

Serotonin is one of the most important neurotransmitters since it is found in many parts of the brain, particularly the cerebral cortex, so it is implicated in most symptoms found in different mental illnesses, especially in our moods and thought processes. Its chemical name is 5-hydroxytryptamine or 5HT, which is used as an abbreviation. Low levels of serotonin are associated with inhibition, emotional instability, impulsivity, aggression, sexual activity, and suicidal behavior. Most of the drugs that are used to treat depression raise the serotonin levels, but in different ways. Too much serotonin, however, is known to have an adverse effect on cardiac functions, so getting the precise amount needed to regulate mood and not cause adverse effects is the challenge to drug manufacturers and psychopharmacologists.

Norepinephrine

Norepinephrine, another important neurotransmitter found at the synaptic cleft, is also known as noradrenalin when it acts as a hormone in the endocrine system. As a neurotransmitter it regulates some of the ANS functions in making sure blood pressure and other bodily functions are elevated and then return to normal during high stress situations. It is also believed to have some implication for panic disorders when it is elevated, although this is probably in concert with the cortical releasing factor (CRF) that also occurs during high stress states and is implicated in PTSD.

Dopamine

Dopamine is similar in structure to norepinephrine and epinephrine. It regulates the motor system that coordinates our movements, so it is important to those with Parkinson's disease where adding dopamine in drugs such as L-dopa may stop or lessen the tremors associated with this disorder. Too much dopamine in the cerebral cortex is associated with the confused thinking of those with schizophrenia, so drugs that block it will reduce some of the positive symptoms. It is associated with exploratory and pleasure-seeking activities. However, we also have learned that dopamine and serotonin may work together so that if there is too much dopamine, serotonin may try to block some of its effects by inhibiting behavior.

GABA

GABA is a neurotransmitter that has an inhibitory effect on neural transmission. It seems to have a major effect on calming down our emotional arousal and reactivity. The benzodiazepine drugs that calm our anxieties work by making the GABA receptor cells more receptive, thus also preventing muscle spasms. Less is known about all the ways that GABA works as compared to the other neurotransmitters, but it is clear that it can reduce anger, hostility, and other negative emotional reactions, too.

DISEASES OF THE BRAIN AND NERVOUS SYSTEM

This section addresses mental illnesses that are caused by damage to the structure and function of this highly complex system.

Delirium

Delirium is a brain syndrome that is characterized by impaired consciousness and cognition. People with delirium appear confused, disoriented and out of touch with their surroundings. They cannot focus and sustain their attention on even the simplest tasks. They have impairments with language and memory. Symptoms come on quickly, within a few hours or day rather than gradually (Table 4.1). They usually subside rather quickly after appropriate treatment. Delirium can be caused by drugs, infections, high fevers, head injury, and other poisons that cross the blood/brain barrier. Sometimes it can leave the person with damage to the brain cells that were involved in the toxic process. Treatment for delirium always involves treatment of the underlying physical disease process as well as treatment of the patient's cognitive symptoms.

Table 4.1. Cardinal Signs and Symptoms: Delirium

- Impairment of consciousness with difficulty focusing, shifting and sustaining attention
- Cognitive impairments including memory, orientation and perception
- Symptoms develop rapidly and vary during the day
- Due to general medical/substance use condition

Dementia

Dementia is a progressively deteriorating disease that typically involves a gradual decline of brain functioning due to a variety of underlying disease processes. Dementia affects judgment, memory, language, and other cognitive processes. It can be caused by stroke, infectious diseases such as West Nile Virus, HIV, syphilis, severe head injury, deteriorating brain diseases such as Parkinson's, Huntington's, and, most commonly, Alzheimer's Disease that affects an estimated 4.5 million Americans. The number of Americans with AD has more than doubled since 1980. Memory impairment is the most common symptom, in addition to *Agnosia* (failure to recognize names, people, and objects), *apraxia* (inability to engage in purposeful acts like buttoning a shirt), *aphasia* (language impairment), and the loss of global intellectual and executive functioning. Genetic factors are strongly implicated in Alzheimer 's disease. While there are no cures for dementia, cognitive slippage may be slowed up to one year in early cases with new medications such as Aricept and Remiryl (Table 4.2).

Amnesic Disorders

Amnesic disorders usually involve the inability of the memory either to record or recall information just learned (Table 4.3). Other cognitive processes may not be impaired. Sometimes it is difficult to tell whether the disorder is part of a dementia. Sometimes the short-term memory disorder is due to medical condition or head trauma. Because of the apparently intact cognitive processes, it is tempting to disbelieve someone with

Table 4.2. Cardinal Signs and Symptoms: Dementia

- Impaired memory
- Inability to learn new information
- Language disturbance (aphasia)
- Impaired ability for motor activities (apraxia)
- Inability to recognize common objects (agnosia)
- Disturbance in planning, organizing, sequencing and abstracting (executive functions)
- Gradual deterioration in functioning from pre-morbid level

Table 4.3. Cardinal Signs and Symptoms: Amnesic Disorder

- Impairment of memory
- Inability to learn new or recall previously learned information
- Memory disturbance does not occur during delirium or dementia
- Due to a general medical/substance use condition

short-term amnesia and, instead, believe the person is malingering. In legal situations, there is self interest to do so and, therefore, psychologists use tests specifically designed to assess for malingering to assist in making this determination. Korsakoff's Disease is a serious amnesic disorder, often the result of chronic alcohol abuse.

Attentional Disorders

Attentional Disorders have become more important in the criminal justice system because more adults are being diagnosed with Adult Attention Deficit Disorders, with or without hyperactivity (ADD and ADHD). We have seen these disorders in children who have learning problems because of impulsivity and difficulties in attention and concentration in school. Most of them are prescribed medication usually a stimulant such as Ritalin (methylphenidate) or Adderall, and sometimes their learning environment is modified to assist them in focusing their attention. We used to think that these brain disorders would be outgrown when the child's brain matured. Now we believe that some of them do not outgrow the disorder, and, rather, the attention and concentration problems and impulsivity follow them into adulthood. These are the people who cannot remember more than one or two items in a sequence, who become restless and agitated if they don't move around, or have such an intense focus on something that they cannot shift their concentration or attention. Interestingly, it does not impact on intelligence even though it does impact their behavior, often making many activities of daily living quite challenging. A new non-stimulant medication called Strattera (atomoxetine) has recently been marketed with some success. In some children and adults, SSRIs and atypical second generation anti-psychotic drugs have been used, although this application has not been approved and is used "off-label."

INTERACTION OF PHYSICAL AND PSYCHOLOGICAL ETIOLOGY

Many of the people we work with in the criminal justice system have multiple disorders that affect their behavior. This may include both organic and non-organic disorders that originate together or develop at different times. For example, a teenager who was without sufficient oxygen to the brain at birth may develop behavior problems that are reinforced by poor discipline. That teenager may then turn to alcohol and other drugs that continue to disinhibit behavior and create more learning deficits. By the end of the teen years that person may become a drug addict and a career criminal, identifying more with the "bad" boy or girl image. This person may even develop psychotic behavior that would probably have occurred whether or not he or she was in trouble with the law. In that case, the teen's alcohol abuse could be seen as self-medication to reduce emotional distress rather than delinquent behavior, or perhaps a combination of both. If arrested, this youth might be bragging to others as a way of covering up perceived inadequacies. If the combined influence on his or her behavior is not readily understood, the youth could be seen simply as malingering, in spite of the fact that he had bona fide psychiatric illness caused by an interaction of physical and psychological influences. Only 20% of youth who are arrested will go on to become a career criminals. The challenge is to identify those who are in that group and intervene early with appropriate mental health treatment in order to lower that number. Mental retardation and other cognitive disorders in youth will be covered in Chapter Twelve.

SUGGESTED READINGS

Beaumont, J. G., Kenealy, P. M., & Rogers, M. J. C. (1999). *The Blackwell Dictionary of neuropsychology*. Oxford: Blackwells

Gazzaniga, M. S., Ivry, R. B., & Mangun, G. R. (1998a). *Cognitive neuroscience: The biology of the mind*. New York: W. W. Norton & Company.

Gazzaniga, M. S., Ivry, R. B., & Mangun, G. R. (1998b). *The working brain: An introduction to neuropsychology*. New York: W. W. Norton & Company.

Mind and brain: Readings from Scientific American (1993). New York: W. H. Freeman and Co.

Parkin, A. J. (1996). *Explorations in cognitive neuropsychology*. Cambridge, MS: Blackwell Publishers.

Pinel, J. P. J. & Edwards, M. (1998). *A colorful introduction to the anatomy of the human brain: A brain and psychology coloring book*. Boston, MA: Allyn & Bacon.

Pinker, S. (1997). *How the mind works*. New York: Penguin.

Posner, M. I. & Raichle, M. E. (1997). *Images of mind*. New York: W. H. Freeman and Company.

Sacks, O. (1990). *The Man Who Mistook His Wife for a Hat and other Clinical Tales*. New York: Harper Perennial.

Thompson, R. F. (1993). *The brain: A neuroscience primer*, (2nd Ed.). New York: W. H. Freeman and Company.

CHAPTER 5

The Psychotic Disorders

SCHIZOPHRENIA

Schizophrenia is undoubtedly the most well known and most severely debilitating of all the psychiatric illnesses known to people. It will typically have devastating impact on the individual, on his or her family and, indirectly, on society and its gatekeepers. The approximate lifetime incidence is 1%, meaning that the risk of any person's developing this disease during his or her lifetime is about one in one hundred. In its 2006 report, the National Institute of Mental Health noted that approximately 2.4 million people 18 years and older will have this disorder in any given year. In 1990, direct and indirect costs were estimated to be $33 billion, accounting for 2.5% of the healthcare dollar. Schizophrenic patients occupy as many as 25% of all hospital beds at any given time. Lost productivity in the United States is estimated to be as high as $20 billion per year, a completed suicide rate at approximately 10%, and premature death from poor self care, substance abuse, poverty and homelessness all represent the tremendous cost of this psychotic disorder.

The general public has many misconceptions about this illness that often lead to increased stigmatization and, for First Responders, ineffective management of afflicted persons whom they encounter in the field. One of the most serious misconceptions is that all persons with schizophrenia are dangerous and violent. The reality is that when properly medicated, treated, and free of alcohol and drugs, persons with this disorder are no more violent or aggressive than anyone else in the general population. A second common belief is that schizophrenic patients have a "split personality." Schizophrenia is a term, literally translated as "split mind." It was coined by a psychiatrist named Eugen Bleuler who was referring to the fact that the schizophrenic's thinking, emotions and behavior are "split" and not integrated, resulting in their often incoherent speech and disorganized behavior. Split personality more accurately describes what we now call Dissociative Identity Disorder or multiple personality disorder.

Schizophrenia is an incredibly heterogeneous disorder that manifests itself in individuals in many different ways. That is, while we agree on a core profile of cardinal signs, symptoms and history, no single patient necessarily manifests all of those characteristics. Some mental health professionals reject the unitary term "schizophrenia" and suggest that it represents many different disorders, referring to them as "the schizophrenias" or schizophrenia spectrum disorders. For most patients, however, the disorder results in fluctuating, gradually deteriorating, or relatively stable disturbances in thinking, behavior, and perception. These disturbances include the presence of "positive" symptoms, such as delusions, hallucinations, and disorganized speech and behavior; and "negative" symptoms, such as poverty of speech, flattened affect, social withdrawal, and avolition. The "positive" symptoms are what we generally understand to represent the "psychotic" state. It is important to understand that while persons diagnosed with this disorder are likely to suffer chronically from schizophrenia, when stabilized they will not be "psychotic." In other words, psychosis is a "state" that is often present in this as well as other serious psychiatric and medical disorders, but it is not synonymous with them. The "negative" symptoms, on the other hand, tend to be more chronic, more difficult to treat and more seriously debilitating in terms of social, occupational and interpersonal functioning.

CLINICAL PICTURE OF SCHIZOPHRENIA

Positive Symptoms

DELUSIONS. A *delusion* is a false, illogical or bizarre belief about the world that has absolutely no basis in reality. We generally associate mental illness with this type of symptom that may reflect paranoid, grandiose, somatic, persecutory or religious themes. Schizophrenic delusions are generally bizarre, meaning that it would be impossible for them to be true. Individuals who believe that their behavior or thoughts are being controlled through electrodes implanted in their brain, that the police officers questioning them are capable of "reading their mind" through radio waves emitted from their brain, that they are Jesus Christ, or that, their intestines are turning to concrete are experiencing bizarre delusions that are often pathonomonic for schizophrenia. First Responders may also encounter individuals who may manifest delusional thinking that is not so obvious to detect without more extensive investigation. Delusions involving beliefs that one is being investigated by the FBI, pursued by drug lords intent on killing the individual, or that one is suffering from an incurable cancer are all possible, although improbable.

HALLUCINATIONS. In contrast to a delusion, a *hallucination* is a false perception of the world in the absence of any physical sensory input.

Hallucinations can involve any of the five sensory modalities although auditory hallucinations are the most characteristic of schizophrenic patients. When patients report false perceptions involving kinesthetic or tactile sensations, olfactory (smell) or even visual hallucinations, the First Responder should consider the possibility that the individual is suffering from an organic or purely physical problem rather than a schizophrenic disorder. Auditory hallucinations often involve voices engaging in a running commentary about the person's behavior, two or more voices arguing or discussing with one another, voices criticizing or taunting the individual or a voice commanding that the person engage in some behavior. Command hallucinations are often potentially dangerous when the voice, often God or the Devil, commands that the individual kill himself or someone else.

Disorganized Speech and Thought

Thinking processes and speech are typically disturbed in persons with schizophrenia. Often, schizophrenia has been described as a "thought disorder" as a result of the fact that these individuals think and reason in ways that appear incoherent, illogical or impossible to understand. First Responders will find that these patients are difficult or impossible to interview. Not only do they lack insight into their difficulties and often deny that they are ill, but they display a variety of characteristic thought disturbances that result in utter confusion for anyone trying to understand them or elicit information. They manifest "loose associations," jumping from topic to topic without any obvious connection of ideas; they engage in "circumstantial and tangential thinking" into which they insert endless irrelevancies and detail into their responses, or they go off precipitously into a train of thought without ever returning to their main point. They may be speaking and suddenly stop or "block" their speech, losing track of their thoughts. Schizophrenic thinking is often very abstract and philosophical, but, in the final analysis, the listener recognizes that no meaning has been communicated. We often refer to this as "poverty of content" or "empty" talk. The very disorganized schizophrenic may make up words (neologisms), refuse to speak at all (mutism), or be totally preoccupied with "invisible forces," for example, witchcraft, sex, religion or philosophy. Remember that many of these signs and symptoms may become chronic, even after the actual psychotic state, characterized particularly by delusions and hallucinations, has remitted or significantly improved. Examples of thought disturbances are provided in Box 5.1.

Behavioral and Emotional Disorganization

First Responders will often recognize individuals with schizophrenia by their strange, inappropriate behavior that inevitably invokes fear and avoidance in the average citizen. Officers will observe these people

---

BOX 5.1

Examples of Disturbances of Thought Processes

Loose Associations and Tangential Thinking

Officer: You seem to be lost in this bus station. Can I help you?

Subject: Yes, thank you officer. I am working here and trying to get a new uniform so I can migrate to the store. They told me to find a better work station so my mother won't be upset and I can... where did you put my dog?

Neologisms

First Responder: The dispatcher has told us that you were complaining of dizziness. Can you tell me what is bothering you?

Subject: I sure can. I can get this noise in my head to die down. The next door neighbors bother me every night with their *audiocerebral injector*. They control my thoughts and I want you to *de-anesthetize* them.

---

engaging in strange mannerisms, gesturing to passersby, pacing in an agitated manner or appearing to talk with an apparently invisible person. At times they may dress inappropriately with heavy clothing during the warmest days, be totally unkempt and disheveled or wear makeup that is excessive and clown-like. Some individuals may assume frozen positions as if they are afraid to move or even be totally immobile, behaviors often described as catatonic immobility.

A person with schizophrenia will often display emotional or affective behaviors that further exaggerate their strange and disturbing presentation. While we ordinarily expect that our emotional tone or affect will match what we are talking about, in schizophrenia this correspondence is often not present. This disconnect or "splitting" is referred to as inappropriate affect and is present when, for instance, the individual cries while describing how much fun they had at a birthday party or laughs in describing how his or her mother was injured by a hit and run driver. Remember that, while many of these characteristics appear in the "schizophrenias," no single person will necessarily manifest all of them, underscoring the heterogeneity of the disorder.

The description of the positive symptoms above is usually associated with the psychotic disorganization that frequently will bring the individual with schizophrenia to the attention of the First Responder. Some patients may initially appear stable but, with the stress of the crisis situation, may later decompensate. It is in this state or the active phase of the illness that persons can be dangerous to themselves and a threat to other citizens or so disabled that they are unable to care for themselves. While this disorganization is often frightening to observe and frequently calls for emergency intervention, surprisingly it is the phase of the illness that is most successfully treated by mental health professionals. Much more insidious and impairing to the person's overall functioning are the negative symptoms that often persist beyond the psychotic episode and may characterize the person's everyday behavior.

Negative Symptoms

Negative symptoms, sometimes referred to as the "defect state," involve characteristics that reflect the absence or insufficiency of normal behavior. Individuals with this disorder will often be quite apathetic and unwilling to engage in everyday activities (*avolition*). They may be uncommunicative or respond to questions with one word and rather impoverished answers (*alogia*). Some individuals will seem to lose their ability to enjoy normal activities and be unable to experience pleasure in what most of us would find fun or enjoyable (*anhedonia*). Many individuals will show no emotion and have a mask like expression despite the content of their speech or how they may be feeling internally. This is referred to as *blunted or flat affect*. All of these symptoms may be less disruptive to personnel who typically face emergent situations in the field, but their influence on the lives of individuals with schizophrenia can be devastating in terms of their inability to work, socialize, and maintain relationships with family and friends. Their presence seems to impact negatively on the likelihood of significant improvement in the individual's disorder and, in contrast to the positive symptoms, the symptoms are very difficult to treat effectively. For a list of Schizophrenic signs and symptoms see Table 5.1.

Classification of Schizophrenia

In order to better understand and treat schizophrenia, clinicians and researchers have developed subtypes of this disorder, each with its distinct signs and symptoms, yet all sharing much of the core clinical picture described above. The fourth edition of the Diagnostic and Statistical Manual of the American Psychiatric Association (DSM-IV-TR) lists five subtypes of schizophrenia: paranoid, disorganized, catatonic, undifferentiated, and residual. *Paranoid* schizophrenics are characterized by prominent delusions and hallucinations of a persecutory or delusional nature, typically without gross disorganization of speech and behavior. The *disorganized* type of schizophrenia, on the other hand, shows gross disorganization of behavior and speech, inappropriate affect and, often, behavior that is silly and childlike. This type shows very little improvement over time, in contrast to the paranoid type that has

Table 5.1. Cardinal Signs and Symptoms: Schizophrenia

- Delusions
- Hallucinations
- Incoherent/Disorganized speech
- Disorganized behavior
- Negative symptoms
- Deterioration of social functioning
- Persistent signs/symptoms for at least 6 months

a better prognosis. Individuals diagnosed with *catatonic* schizophrenia typically display a variety of movement disorders including stupor, waxy flexibility where they maintain fixed postures for long periods, facial grimacing, or periods of agitated and at times violent behavior. *Undifferentiated* schizophrenia is a subtype reserved for individuals who are clearly suffering from the disorder but who do not fit into any other type. Finally, persons who have had at least one episode of schizophrenia, but who do not manifest any of the major psychotic symptoms described above, may be diagnosed with *residual* schizophrenia.

Readers should keep in mind that, while these subtypes may have some research or clinical value, most individuals with this disorder will display many combinations of symptoms at different stages of their illness and be very difficult to place neatly into any single category.

Risk, Prognostic, Demographic and Cultural Factors

The risk of anyone developing schizophrenia at some time in his or her lifetime is 1%, a statistic that holds both nationally and internationally. While the risk is generally the same for both sexes, males develop the disorder earlier, typically between 18 and 25, while the average age of onset for woman is from 26 to 45 years old. Rarely does anyone develop this disorder after the age of 45. Women generally respond better to antipsychotic medication and have better overall treatment outcomes than men as the disorder progresses. While the diagnosis of schizophrenia has been more common in poor or devalued ethnic minorities, the increased rate in these cultural groups is more likely an artifact of bias and cultural stereotyping.

Historically, the mental health community in concert with the general population has maintained a pessimistic view regarding the prognosis for positive outcomes in schizophrenia. While the overall picture suggests that most individuals with the disorder will struggle with moderate to severe levels of impairment throughout their lives, some longitudinal research suggests some variability in outcomes. In 1991, Leff and his colleagues studied patients with schizophrenia who had been hospitalized around the world. They found that, on a 5 year follow-up after discharge, 17% of the patients had experienced full remission of their symptoms with no further psychotic episodes; 13% had partial remission with no further episodes; 15% experienced further episodes but enjoyed full remission between episodes; 33% had further episodes without full remission; and 19% had continuation of their initial psychotic episode without remission over the 5 year period. Judging from these data, the outlook for patients with this disorder may not be as pessimistic as we once believed.

Etiology of Schizophrenia

The causes of schizophrenia are highly complex and multidimensional, leaving researchers the task of piecing together an intricate puzzle involving genetic, biological, and psychosocial contributions. The fact that we often refer to the disorder as "the schizophrenias" suggests that contemporary researchers and clinicians conceptualize it as a broad syndrome manifested by a diverse set of genetically based brain disorders primarily involving brain neurochemistry and neuroanatomy and intrauterine events that may be precipitated or exacerbated by psychological or social stressors. These factors will be discussed below.

Researchers agree that genes are significantly involved in rendering some individuals vulnerable to schizophrenia. While the mode of transmission is unclear, it is generally agreed that not one but many genes combine to raise the threshold of this vulnerability. Genetic researchers have established this heritability through family, adoption, and twin studies that point unequivocally to the presence of this vulnerability. Family studies involve identifying the risk of developing schizophrenia when first degree biological relatives suffer from the illness. Relative risks, for instance, of an individual developing the disorder when one or both parents are schizophrenic are about 12 and 48%, respectively. If one sibling is schizophrenic, the risk is approximately 15%. The problem with this type of family study is that it does not take into consideration the role that environment has on the development of the disorder. The question becomes, "Does living in the same environment with your parents or siblings cause the disorder or are genes responsible?" To address this question, researchers rely on other research methods including adoption and twin studies.

Adoption studies strive to remove the issue of environmental effects from the genetic contribution. Individuals who have been adopted, raised apart from their biological parents who have been diagnosed with schizophrenia, and who develop the disorder are compared with normal control adoptees whose parents did not have schizophrenia. The general findings of these adoption studies conclude that children raised apart from their schizophrenic parent(s) have a higher average rate of developing the disorder than control adoptees, even though their adopted families did not have the disorder.

Perhaps the most compelling evidence of genetic vulnerability comes from twin studies with identical or fraternal twins who share 100 and 50% of their genes, respectively. In these studies, if one identical twin develops schizophrenia, there is nearly a 50% chance that the other twin will also develop the disorder. Concordance rates for fraternal twins, who share only 50% of their genes, is about 17%. One would reason that if environment were primarily responsible for development of the disorder that the rates of identical vs. fraternal twins who have been raised together would not differ. On the other hand, if genetic heritability were primary, we would expect identical twins to share schizophrenia 100% of the time and fraternal twins to share it 50% of the time. When we consider that the average risk of developing the disorder in the general population is 1%, it is clear from these studies that genetics plays a major role in the development of schizophrenia. However, it is also evident from our research that genes do not account for the entire etiological picture. Other factors must play a role in the development of the disorder.

Several theories involving potential markers for schizophrenia, prenatal and perinatal factors, and neuroanatomical features have been proposed, some with little empirical validation. One area involves smooth-pursuit eye movement that enables one to track objects smoothly across a visual plane. Impairment in this ability has been found among many individuals diagnosed with schizophrenia as well as in their family members. Attentional deficits have also been identified that can be measured by specific visual testing and, like eye tracking dysfunction, can serve as a marker for schizophrenia that may be linked to a specific gene. By identifying these *markers*, scientists can look for associated genes that provide further clues to the etiology of the disorder.

Another interesting, but unproven, theory involves the findings that schizophrenics have a high likelihood of being born in the winter or early spring months suggesting some intrauterine insult may arise from a viral etiology. While some research has pointed to prenatal and intrauterine exposure to influenza and a high incidence of birth complications in schizophrenics, there is limited evidence of a virus connected to schizophrenia.

Neuroanatomical research studying the brains of individuals with schizophrenia rather consistently points to the presence of enlarged ventricles in many, but not all, schizophrenics. As you read in the previous chapter, ventricles are large, fluid filled spaces in the brain. This enlargement appears more common in men than women, seems proportional to the duration of the illness, and is associated with those individuals who manifest significant negative symptoms, suggesting more cognitive impairment. In addition to ventricular abnormalities, PET scans have revealed an underactivity in the pre-frontal lobes of schizophrenic patients when compared to normals. The frontal lobes are largely responsible for our higher order abstract thinking and may also be associated with the negative symptoms of schizophrenia like amotivation and avolition. Neuroanatomical factors are likely to be implicated in the cognitive impairment of persons with schizophrenia and involve multiple sites in the brain. The brain damage may begin prenatally and develop insidiously, long before the individual develops a full blown schizophrenic episode.

No area of research has yielded more interest or translated into such major treatment advances than that involving the neurochemistry of the brain. As discussed earlier, one very popular theory of schizophrenia causation involves the role of dopamine, one of the neurosynaptic transmitters. The theory suggests that excessive dopamine activity at certain pathways in the brain results in what we call schizophrenic or psychotic behavior. Empirical support for this involves several facts. Psychotropic drugs that are known to partially block the metabolism of dopamine are often effective in reducing schizophrenic-like behavior. In some patients the negative side effect of these anti-psychotic drugs is to produce symptoms similar to Parkinson's disease, the etiology of which is related to insufficient dopamine. Researchers have also found that in the treatment of Parkinson's disease with a dopamine medication called L-dopa, some patients develop psychotic symptoms. Finally, long-term use of amphetamines and cocaine can also increase levels of dopamine in the brain and produce paranoid psychotic symptoms in many individuals.

While this evidence is certainly very supportive, it is by no means conclusive. Many patients treated with dopamine blocking medication are not helped since some of these medications have little effect on the negative symptoms of schizophrenia. When these dopamine blocking agents are used to treat psychotic episodes precipitated by toxic substances, medical illnesses, depression or bipolar disorder, they tend to be equally effective, suggesting the effects of dopamine blockage are not specific to schizophrenia. Regardless, there is no question that dopamine as well as other neurosynaptic transmitters, including serotonin, is involved with this disorder, but in a highly complex fashion that researchers are only beginning to uncover.

The final piece of the complicated puzzle involving causes of schizophrenia includes psychological and social factors that are sometimes listed under the general term "stress." While current theories of causation do not suggest that psychosocial stress alone is responsible for this disorder, many emphasize the role that such factors may play in contributing to or exacerbating the illness.

Psychoanalytically oriented theories of schizophrenia dating back to Sigmund Freud emphasized early life experiences related to parenting and trauma in explaining the cause of schizophrenia. Schizophrenogenic mothers characterized as cold, rejecting and domineering, as well as "double-binding" family members whose confusing communications left the child in a helpless, "no-win" situation, were described as the culprit in the etiology of the disorder. While there is little argument that these types of relationships and experiences are stressful and may inevitably result in psychological distress, researchers today do not suggest that such factors cause schizophrenia.

A more fruitful line of research has developed around how certain family emotional environments increase the likelihood of relapse in patients already suffering from this illness. Research has shown that individuals with families that demonstrate high levels of criticism, hostility and dissatisfaction with them have a much higher risk of relapse than those where these conditions do not exist. This constellation of factors is called Expressed Emotion (EE) and research in one study (Butzlaf and Hooley, 1998) demonstrated patient relapse rates of 65% and 35% in families with high and low EE, respectively. This line of research is valuable in guiding our treatment and interventions with families and individuals diagnosed with schizophrenia.

In summary, we see that the etiological factors in schizophrenia are many and highly complex, combining genetic, biological and psychosocial factors. Researchers and clinicians have come to describe this interplay as representing the "diathesis-stress" model of causation in which inherited vulnerability combined with stressful circumstances results in the development of overt schizophrenia.

Treatment Approaches

Treatment approaches to schizophrenia over the years have varied according to our understanding of its causes. Primitive cultures exorcised demons who were seen as inhabiting the deranged person and even drilled holes in their heads to allow the demons to escape. More enlightened approaches were developed in the nineteenth and twentieth centuries as physicians realized the biological bases for serious mental illnesses like schizophrenia. However, even these approaches have turned out to be naïve and, in some cases, very destructive. Insulin shock therapy, prefrontal lobotomies, and electroconvulsive therapy were used, often indiscriminately even up to the 1960s, to treat people with schizophrenia.

Current treatment regimes typically include psychotropic medications combined with a variety of psychological and social interventions that are designed to help the patient avoid deterioration in their functioning and to live productive and fulfilling lives.

The introduction of neuroleptic drugs like Thorazine, Haldol and Mellaril in the early 1950s brought about a revolution in the treatment of this disorder. These drugs were seen as blocking the neurosynaptic transmitter dopamine in the brain, thus reducing the very disturbing positive symptoms of schizophrenia including hallucinations and delusions. While these drugs have reduced the presence of these symptoms in up to 60% of patients, they by no means represent a "cure" of the disorder. Many patients do not benefit from the medication, and some of the earlier medications had little impact on the negative symptoms. Newer drugs, called *atypical anti-psychotics* are more effective in reducing symptoms and cause fewer uncomfortable side effects. Most recently, combinations of second line atypicals, small doses of first line anti-psychotics, and mood stabilizers are used to reduce the various symptoms of schizophrenia and have a lower side effects profile than the earlier use of large doses of anti-psychotic medication alone. See Box 3.4 for a list of the most popular antipsychotic medications used today.

Unpleasant side effects from the medication are one of the major reasons why many patients relapse and need to be readmitted to a psychiatric hospital. Anti-psychotic drugs often result in excessive sedation, blurred vision, expressionless face, disturbed motor functioning and strange facial movements including the protruding of the tongue, lip smacking and puffing of the cheeks. Sometimes these physical symptoms are mistaken for signs of schizophrenia rather than the result of drug treatment. Newer drugs tend to minimize these problems.

While treatment with psychotropic drugs are the centerpiece in the treatment of schizophrenia, psychosocial interventions including social skills training, vocational rehabilitation, supportive employment and housing alternatives, as well as effective case management, all play a critical role in maximizing each individual's potential to live a full and productive life. Social skills training addresses the negative symptoms of the disorder and teaches the person ways to converse with others, to maintain eye contact and to maintain interpersonal relationships. First Responders will be faced with the homeless population in many communities, many of whom suffer from serious and persistent mental illness as well as substance abuse disorders. Communities that provide resources for supported housing and vocational training can reduce those numbers, and gatekeepers in law enforcement can be helpful in identifying those most amenable to help.

The days of long-term hospitalization that deprived persons with serious mental illness of their coping skills and self-esteem, and too often simply warehoused them, have slowly given way to supportive community environments where individuals learn to cope with stress more effectively, reducing the likelihood of decompensation and rehospitalization. Gradually, the philosophy surrounding the management of schizophrenia has focused on the empowerment of patients to be involved in their own recovery process. Persons with this disorder have the same needs, hopes and aspirations, along with the same stresses and strains of life, as any other individual. They differ in that their illness impairs their fundamental abilities to accurately perceive, cope with, and solve these everyday life problems. However, the combination of psychosocial interventions, family education and support, solid community support systems for housing and employment, with appropriate drug therapy, can enable individuals with schizophrenia to manage these problems more effectively and to live productive lives.

Children and Schizophrenia

Some small percentage of children (0.2%) do have the onset of schizophrenia, usually in their mid to late teen years, although a small number may show signs even earlier. Some of these youth begin to use drugs in an attempt to self-medicate the symptoms of their developing schizophrenias. Often the diagnosis is confused with reports of hallucinations or delusions that may be attributed to their substance abuse rather than the schizophrenic process. However, if diagnosed early enough, it is possible to teach them how to manage their disorder in a way similar to those with adult onset of schizophrenia. This includes finding the appropriate medication and adding others if there are also symptoms of emotional dysregulation and aggression. Additionally, treatment involves teaching teenagers how to take responsibility for their own mental health needs, including reducing environmental stressors in their lives. Sometimes individual or family therapy is also recommended especially when social skills, speech and language deficits, and family dysfunction require intervention.

OTHER PSYCHOTIC DISORDERS

As we discussed in Chapter Three, the Diagnostic and Statistical Manual of the American Psychiatric Association, Fourth Edition lists several other psychotic disorders in its classification system. Three of those diagnoses are of particular importance to First Responders. Delusional Disorder, Brief Psychotic Disorder and Schizoaffective Disorder are characterized by delusions, hallucinations and/or mood symptoms similar in some ways to schizophrenia, but are clearly distinct entities. Keep in mind that the psychotic state is not unique to schizophrenia, but also occurs in other disorders. These disorders have their unique characteristics that the First Responder can learn to identify.

Delusional Disorder

Delusional Disorder is characterized by the presence of false beliefs about the world that we refer to as delusions. Delusional Disorder, which is relatively rare, can be differentiated from schizophrenia by the absence of other symptoms, including the negative or defect state, as well as very disorganized, catatonic speech or behavior. The delusions in this disorder usually are not bizarre as they typically are in schizophrenia. That is, the delusions could in reality be possible, but, in fact, are not. A police officer may encounter an individual who reports that he is a drug informant being followed by a gang member who wants to kill him. While such a situation might be true and possible, in this case it is the result of a paranoid delusion. Other delusions may revolve around themes of grandiosity, jealousy, or undying love. For instance, stalkers may suffer from Delusional Disorder, believing that the individuals they pursue truly love and want them. Somatic delusions also exist in which individuals believe that they suffer from some physical illness or defect.

Patients with Delusional Disorder may have relatively unaffected lives outside the influence of their delusion and may not seek treatment or, depending on the type of delusion they experience, may not come to the attention of a First Responder. A law enforcement officer may respond to a domestic violence call and discover an irate husband accusing his wife of infidelity. After investigating the incident, the officer may discover that this is a case of Delusional Disorder given that there is absolutely no basis for the accusation and the husband is intractable in his jealous belief. However, the officer may also discover that, remarkably, the subject is a successful and respected businessman in the community who manifests no other emotional impairments. Individuals with other types of delusions may suffer more disability, but typically much less than in schizophrenia. Relevant criteria for Delusional Disorder are provided in Table 5.2.

There are a number of circumstances where the individual suffering from Delusional Disorder will have a greater likelihood of coming into

Table 5.2. Cardinal Signs and Symptoms: Delusional Disorder

- Non bizarre delusions (i.e., jealousy, grandiose)
- Behavior and speech are not odd/bizarre
- No marked impairment in functioning
- No history of schizophrenia
- No significant mood disorder

Table 5.3. Cardinal Signs and Symptoms: Brief Psychotic Disorder

- Delusions
- Hallucinations
- Disorganized speech/behavior
- Duration is from 1 day to 1 month
- Patient eventually returns to premorbid functioning

contact with the legal system. One example involves the patient's reaction to being labeled "legally incompetent." Given that an individual manifests delusional thinking, particularly of the persecutory type, family and friends may respond by initiating action to have the person declared incompetent to handle his or her affairs. The delusional patient predictably will perceive this action as a confirmation of their distorted beliefs. Often they will react with hostility or initiate legal action themselves. The possibility of physical violence fueled by paranoid and persecutory beliefs always remains a concern for the community.

Paranoid individuals are frequently seen as quite litigious and will often engage the legal system in pursuing complaints of harassment and unfair practices by others. Those people with the paranoid type of Delusional Disorder may initially present as emotionally intact, unlike their paranoid schizophrenic counterparts, and be taken quite seriously. These individuals may engage attorneys in frivolous lawsuits or the police in investigating noise complaints by neighbors, unfair labor practices, or property rights issues all arising, they assert, from the malevolent motivations of others who wish to persecute them.

Brief Psychotic Disorder

Brief Psychotic Disorder involves the presence of delusions, hallucinations or other positive symptoms including disorganized speech and or behavior. These symptoms are typically acute and last anywhere from one day to one month with return to normal state within that period. Often these symptoms are precipitated by highly stressful or traumatic situations that overwhelm an individual's ability to cope. First Responders who deal with serious accidents, fires, and catastrophic events may encounter individuals suffering from this disorder. During

> **BOX 5.2**
>
> **Operational Factors for First Responders**
>
> - The psychotic subject is likely to be extremely fearful and vulnerable.
> - Distrust and paranoia tend to be common and, in their defense, subjects may be potentially violent.
> - First Responders should approach the subject in a non threatening manner with no unnecessary show of force.
> - Minimize stress and sensory overload for the psychotic person who is already overwhelmed by internal stimuli (hallucinations/delusions) by speaking softly and eliminating unnecessary personnel or equipment.
> - Do not challenge the subject's delusional thinking; listen carefully, empathizing with his/her concerns.
> - Offer assistance initially by asking the subject what might be helpful to him/her.
> - Evaluate the situation including the possibility that drugs may be involved, and offer the psychotic subject your plan in a firm manner.

this psychotic episode, it is difficult or impossible to differentiate it from schizophrenia or other psychotic disorders without understanding the person's history, time of onset, and precipitating factors. The fact is that the disorder must resolve within a relatively short time and not be accompanied by other symptoms and the functional decline characteristic of schizophrenia. See Table 5.3 for cardinal signs and symptoms of Brief Psychotic Disorder.

Schizoaffective Disorder

Schizoaffective Disorder was introduced in the Diagnostic and Statistical Manual as a disorder incorporating both the active phase of schizophrenia with the symptoms of a mood disorder. It remains a relatively controversial diagnosis and one that is often difficult to differentiate from schizophrenia. It is not uncommon for patients suffering from schizophrenia to experience episodes of depression concurrently with their hallucinations or delusions. However, a schizoaffective diagnosis can only be made when these symptom clusters occur concurrently and, at some time during the illness, there is at least a two week period in which the individual has psychotic symptoms in the absence of any mood symptoms. The treatment and prognosis for this disorder are basically the same as for schizophrenia with the addition of medication to address the mood symptoms.

Finally, it cannot be emphasized enough that psychotic episodes occur in a variety of different disorders with very different causes. Before considering any of the disorders discussed in this chapter, it is critical that we rule out causes from substances like amphetamines, alcohol and cocaine as well as a variety of physical illnesses from dementia to cancer. It follows that if such underlying causes are discovered, the treatment approaches utilized will be vastly different. Treating an individual who is psychotic as a result of brain tumor with interventions appropriate for schizophrenic patients would be unsuccessful and dangerous.

Operational factors useful for the First Responder in dealing with psychotic subjects are described in Box 5.2.

SUGGESTED READINGS

Birchwood, M. J. (1989). *Schizophrenia: An integrated approach to research and treatment.* New York: New York University Press.

Brown, M. J. & Roberts, D. P. (2000). *Growing up with a schizophrenic mother.* Jefferson, NC: McFarland.

Cromwell, R. L. & Synder, C. R. (Eds.). (1993). *Schizophrenia: origins, processes, treatment, and outcome.* New York: Oxford University Press.

Gottesman, I. L. (1991). *Schizophrenia genesis: The origins of madness.* New York: W.H. Freeman.

Green, M. F. (2001). *Schizophrenia revealed: From neurons to social interactions.* New York: W.W. Norton.

Hatfield, A. B. & Lefly, H. P. (1993). *Surviving mental illness: Stress, coping and adaptation.* New York: Guilford.

Heinrichs, R. W. (2001). *In search of madness: Schizophrenia and neuroscience.* New York: Oxford University Press.

Johnson, E. C., Humphreys, M. S., Lang, F. H., Lawrie, S. M., & Sandler, R. (1999). *Schizophrenia: Concepts and clinical management.* New York: Cambridge University Press.

Keefe, R. & Harvey, P. D. (1994). *Understanding schizophrenia: A guide to the new research on causes and treatment.* New York: Free Press.

Lidz, T. (1985). *Schizophrenia and the family.* New York: International Universities Press.

Miller, R. & Mason, S. E. (Eds.). (2002). *Diagnosis: Schizophrenia.* New York: Columbia University Press.

Monahan, J. & Steadman, H. J. (Eds.). (1994). *Violence and mental disorder.* Chicago: University of Chicago Press.

Munro, A. (1999). *Delusional Disorder.* New York: Cambridge University Press.

Oltmanns, T. F. & Maher, B. A. (Eds.). (1988). *Delusional beliefs.* New York: John Wiley.

Straube, E. R. & Hahlweg, K. (1990). *Schizophrenia: Concepts, vulnerability, and intervention.* New York: Springer-Verlag.

Torrey, E. F. (1995). *Surviving schizophrenia: A manual for families, consumers, and providers.* New York: Harper.

Torrey, E. F. (2006). *Surviving schizophrenia: A manual for families, patients and providers* (5th Ed.). Quill Publishers.

White, G. L. & Mullen, P. E. (1989). *Jealousy: Theory, research and clinical strategies.* New York: Guilford Press.

CHAPTER 6

The Mood Disorders

Our mood involves a pervasive and sustained emotion that colors our perceptions of the world. We feel sadness and joy, anger and anxiety in reaction to our interaction with others, to successes and failures we experience, and in reaction to our internal, psychological self explorations. Emotions like sadness and joy occur as part of everyday life and occur in reaction to normal life events such as the loss of loved ones, failures and disappointments as well as successes that all of us encounter at some time in our lives. First Responders who face life and death situations on a daily basis are at risk for exaggerated emotional reactions after involvement in a shooting incident, after witnessing catastrophic accidents, or after losing a victim that they have tried to save. Grief or mild depressive reactions in these situations may result in feelings of guilt, sadness, sleeplessness and restlessness that are quite predictable and likely to resolve quickly. We may experience the "blues," feeling "bummed out" or simply "down" in response to some conflict or frustration in our lives or in reaction to a holiday or anniversary that ignites memories of an earlier sad or traumatic time. All of these reactions and emotions, including sadness and joy, are quite normal and universal and do not usually result in a clinical mood disorder. However, when these mood states are exaggerated, persistent and recurrent, when they occur in the absence of any environmental event or stressor, and/or result in significant social, occupational or interpersonal impairment, they rise to the level of a clinical and diagnosable disorder.

The Diagnostic and Statistical Manual of the American Psychiatric Association, Fourth Edition (DSM-IV-TR) lists five major mood disorders including Major Depressive Disorder, Dysthymic Disorder, Bipolar I and II Disorders and Cyclothymic Disorder. These categories are in addition to depression and mania that are the direct result of certain substances or a general medical condition. Clinical mood disorders, particularly depression, which are likely to require attention from a professional, affect approximately 20% of women and 10% of men during their lifetime. According to a report issued by the National Institute of

Mental Health issued in 2006 approximately 20.9 million American adults, or about 9.5% of the U.S. population age 18 and older in a given year, have a mood disorder. Depressive disorders, the "common cold" of psychiatric illness, typically begin in the 20s, 30s or 40s, and, according to the National Institute, Major Depressive Disorder is the leading cause of disability in the United States for ages 15 to 44, affecting approximately 14.8 million American adults, or about 6.7% of the U.S. population age 18 and older in a given year. Bipolar disorder, formerly called manic-depressive illness, begins much earlier, in the late teens and twenties, and has been reported to affect about 1% of the population at some time in their lives with no difference in prevalence between men and women. Sex is a major demographic risk factor for depression, but social class, race, and culture appear unrelated. Bipolar disorder, however, tends to be diagnosed more commonly in upper socioeconomic classes, although this may be an artifact of diagnostic biases or cultural prejudice.

MAJOR DEPRESSIVE DISORDER

The most serious and debilitating depression is called *Major Depressive Disorder* (MDD). Persons suffering from MDD complain of pervasive feelings of sadness and depression that last for a minimum of two weeks and result in significant impairment in daily functioning. They experience feelings of worthlessness, hopelessness, and guilt as well as frequent crying spells, accompanied by cognitive impairments including concentration difficulties and inability to make decisions. A central feature of serious depression is the inability to experience pleasure from life called *anhedonia*. Depressed individuals often withdraw from relationships with others, avoid work, and lose all motivation, drive, and will to live. In addition to emotional and cognitive involvement, depressive symptoms include many physical problems called *neurovegetative signs*. Sleep, appetite and sexual disturbances are common, along with fatigue and total loss of energy. Some depressed individuals will experience insomnia and disturbed sleep patterns as well as decreased appetite and weight loss. Others will experience just the reverse with insatiable need to eat and retreat to the bed where they vegetate and sleep constantly. Perhaps the most distressing symptom that the First Responder may encounter is the person's preoccupation with death and thoughts and/or plans of suicide. This problem will be discussed more fully below.

Some individuals with more severe depressions may experience psychotic symptoms during a depressive episode with hallucinations (false perceptions) and/or delusions (false beliefs). Patients may hear God condemning them for their grave sins or insist that they suffer from poverty when, in fact, they are financially well off. These

Table 6.1. Cardinal Signs and Symptoms: Major Depressive Episode

- Depressed mood
- Loss of pleasure in all activities
- Appetite and sleep disturbance
- Psychomotor agitation or retardation
- Fatigue
- Guilt
- Cognitive impairments (i.e. concentration, memory)
- Suicidal thoughts
- Impairment in daily functioning
- Signs and symptoms for at least 2 weeks

psychotic features occur in 5 to 15% of depressions and suggest a poorer response to treatment. When individuals experience these symptoms in a depressive episode, they are likely to experience a reoccurrence in all future episodes.

In describing mood disorders, including MDD, clinicians and researchers refer to the disorder in terms of episodes with an identifiable beginning and end. The average untreated episode of MDD typically lasts between 6 and 9 months. When it first occurs usually between 25 and 30 years old, we refer to it as MDD, Single Episode. Approximately 70 to 80% of all single episode cases will experience a second occurrence and qualify for a diagnosis of Major Depressive Disorder, Recurrent (Table 6.1). Between episodes, after successful treatment, the individual may function quite well and at first glance, it would not necessarily be recognized that the person had any difficulties. Interepisodic functioning, however, is quite variable and some people will suffer chronically from some level of mood disturbance.

DYSTHYMIC DISORDER

Another milder form of depression is called *Dysthymic Disorder* (Table 6.2). This is considered a chronic condition in which the mood problems last a minimum of 2 years with no relief for more than two months at a time. The symptoms are qualitatively the same as in major depression but are not as severe and do not include psychotic episodes, anhedonia, or suicidal preoccupation. Having dysthymic disorder does not guarantee that individuals will not at some point develop a major depressive episode. In those cases we refer to the clinical picture as "double depression."

Table 6.2. Cardinal Signs and Symptoms: Dysthymic Disorder

- Depressed mood
- Sleep and appetite disturbance
- Fatigue/low energy
- Low self esteem
- Cognitive impairments
- Feelings of hopelessness
- Impairment in daily functioning
- Signs and symptoms for at least 2 years

BIPOLAR DISORDERS

Major depression and Dysthymia are often referred to as unipolar mood disorders in contrast to bipolar disorders in which the individual may cycle between different mood states. Once referred to as manic-depressive illness, *Bipolar Disorder* is characterized by shifts in mood between serious depression and mania, in which the individual experiences feelings of elation, grandiosity, expansiveness or irritability. When encountering an individual experiencing a manic episode, you are likely to see someone who is extremely talkative, has racing thoughts, and engages in behaviors that are highly pleasure-seeking, including gambling, spending sprees, excessive and indiscriminate sexuality, all of which represents extremely poor judgment. Individuals suffering from mania do not typically feel a need for sleep and are highly distractible. It is difficult to stop or derail them from their activities. Some people in a manic state engage in criminal behavior, fueled by their need for immediate gratification, expansive feelings that they can do no wrong, and their overwhelming poor judgment. In some cases individuals may be so disorganized that they experience delusions and or hallucinations (Table 6.3).

The *DSM-IV-TR* recognizes three major types of bipolar spectrum disorders: *Bipolar I*, *Bipolar II*, and *Cyclothymic Disorders*. In all three, individuals will at some point in the course of their illness experience both depressed and elevated or irritable moods. These differ primarily in the severity of the symptoms as well as the degree of impairment in functioning the persons may suffer. Bipolar I disorder requires that individuals must have at least one manic episode at some point in the course of their lives and that this episode must last one week or more. Even if the person never has another manic episode or all future episodes involve major depression, the diagnosis remains the same. Bipolar II involves the presence of major depressive episodes in addition to at least one hypomanic episode. A hypomanic episode is similar to a manic episode, but is less severe, involves no impairment of functioning or psychotic symptoms, and must last at least four days. According to the

Table 6.3. Cardinal Signs and Symptoms: Bipolar I Disorder, Manic Episode

---

- Inflated self esteem or grandiosity
- Decreased need for sleep
- Highly talkative
- Racing thoughts
- Distractibility
- Increased activity level
- Psychomotor agitation
- Excessive involvement in pleasurable activities with probability of negative consequences

---

DSM-IV-TR, no manic episode can occur in Bipolar II disorder. Finally, Cyclothymic disorder is characterized by numerous mild depressed and hypomanic episodes that persist for at least 2 years with no history of the more severe manic or major depressive episodes. We may describe an individual with Cyclothymic disorder as "moody" with no extended periods in which they experienced "normal" or euthymic mood. Many individuals with cyclothymia will go on to develop a full blown bipolar disorder at some point in their lives.

As in Major Depressive disorder, the bipolar spectrum of disorders occur in discrete episodes that may include major depression, mania, hypomania, or a mixed state in which the individual experiences alternating manic and severe depressive symptoms, all during the same episode. In between these discrete episodes, the person's functioning may range from optimal to severely impaired. For the episode to be considered discrete, the individual must be symptom free for at least two months before another episode.

The average age of onset for bipolar disorder is about 20 years old, with few developing the disorder after the age of 40. It is known that some medication prescribed for depression, including SSRI's described in Chapter Three, can trigger a manic episode changing the mood from depression to mania. The course of the disorder tends to be chronic with alternating periods of depression and mania. Suicide attempts are a major risk in bipolar disorder in an estimated 20% of those diagnosed.

ETIOLOGY OF MOOD DISORDERS

The causes of mood disorders are varied and typically involve a complex interplay of biological, psychological, and social factors that can produce a variant along the spectrum of mood problems ranging from situational and transient sadness to major depression and mania with psychotic features. Each of these major etiological factors will be discussed below.

Biological Factors

As we saw in the schizophrenia and the psychotic disorders, genetic predisposition plays a very important role. Research utilizing family, adoption, and twin studies has consistently found that mood disorders occur more frequently in relatives of mood disordered persons than in the general population. Most convincing are twin studies where scientists evaluate the frequency with which monozygotic twins with 100% of the same genetic makeup have the disorder, compared to dizogotic twins who share 50% of their genes. The theory states that, if genetic factors are critical, then the disorder should be present in identical twins significantly more frequently than in fraternal twins. Most studies confirm this notion. Data from several studies indicate that if one twin has a mood disorder, an identical twin has up to three times more risk of developing a mood disorder than a fraternal twin. In one study the risk of an identical twin developing major depression when the co-twin suffered from the illness was 60% and 14% for fraternal twins. The risks for bipolar disorder are even higher.

The accumulation of research on the genetics of mood disorders suggests that the more severe the disorder, the greater the genetic contribution; that genes play a less central role in causation for men than for women; that there is no single gene responsible for mood disorders, and that the likelihood is that they result from the cumulative effect of many genes combined with many environmental factors and precipitants. There is no question that while genetic factors are important contributors to mood disorders, other biological, environmental and social factors play central roles in both the etiology of mood disorders and in the specific forms in which they are expressed. It has been estimated that between 60 and 80% of the causes of depression are psychological in nature.

The area of biological research into mood disorders that has received more attention in recent years is the study of brain neurochemistry and the role of neurotransmitter systems. Initially referred to as the "catecholamine hypothesis," the theory holds that the depletion of certain chemicals, for instance norepinephrine, at critical synaptic sites in the brain contributed to chemical dysregulation resulting in disordered mood states. More recently, clinical researchers have suggested that the transmitter serotonin regulates mood reactions, and, when its level is depleted, other transmitters including norepinephrine and dopamine become dysregulated resulting in mood impairments. Administration of antidepressant medication addresses this chemical dysregulation by making these neurotransmitters more available in certain pathways of the brain.

Psychological and Environmental Factors

Law enforcement personnel, firefighters, paramedics and other First Responders face traumatic situations on a daily basis. Not only do they deal with victims who are in crisis, traumatized by crime, natural disaster and illness, but they themselves face the chronic stress of dealing with and taking responsibility for intervening in these crises. The predictable result of this precipitating stress for both the professional as well as the victim is psychological disequilibrium, often in the form of depression. We realize, however, that stress of many types is part of everyday life. Job stress, long hours, marital conflicts, death of loved ones, disappointments, illness, and losses in all areas of life contribute to changes in our mood. For most First Responders and civilians, fortunately, such stressors are handled without serious psychological problems, and emotional symptoms are brief and uncomplicated. For a significant number of individuals who face these same stressors, however, serious depression, bipolar disorder, or other mental illness may result. In order to explain this difference, we must recall that some individuals are vulnerable to mood disorders by virtue of their genetic as well as their psychological makeup. When such a vulnerable individual is faced with a significant environmental stressor, the interaction among these factors may result in a mood disorder. This formulation is often referred to as the *diathesis-stress model.*

Vulnerability to mood disorders is not associated solely with biological influences. Psychological vulnerabilities develop as a consequence of individuals' developmental history and the unique constellation of life events and learning experiences they have accumulated. One influential clinical researcher, Aaron Beck, has theorized that people's unique manner of perceiving the world, themselves, and the future is developed early in childhood. Beck's cognitive theory of depression suggests that when children experience many negative events early in their lives, for instance, constant criticism, physical or sexual abuse, or deaths of significant others, they develop a negative schema, framework or belief system in those areas that will affect their ability to think logically about similar situations in the future and render them at risk for depression. For example, an experienced paramedic who on one occasion does not begin CPR quickly enough on a victim, begins to believe she is incompetent based on this failure and ultimately experiences a major depressive disorder. Assuming she learned from chronically demeaning and critical parents to blame herself for any mistake, Beck would say she had developed a negative schema that was elicited by any mistake she might make. This schema resulted in her automatic thought that she was "worthless and incompetent" and, finally, in her depression. Cognitive theory also describes cognitive errors that people vulnerable to depression may develop, including overgeneralization ("One mistake means I'm incompetent") and black and white thinking ("If I am not perfect, I am worthless"). Most research in cognitive theory supports the notion that depression is highly correlated to negative, pessimistic cognitions.

Another eminent researcher, Martin Seligman, experimented with dogs and rats and discovered that they were able to function well when they could avoid occasional shocks administered to them by pressing a lever. However, when the shocks were administered on a random and variable basis and nothing they did allowed them to avoid them, these animals became listless, stopped trying, and basically developed "depression." Seligman applied this theory to humans and described it as "learned helplessness." Thus, when we find that all our efforts to cope with life problems are fruitless, the theory suggests that we begin to perceive situations as hopeless and that our inability to cope is our fault. This sense of helplessness becomes pervasive and is stable across all life stressors we face, leaving us chronically vulnerable to depression as well as anxiety. Consider a woman who has been chronically victimized by a physically and psychologically abusive husband or partner. She told daily that she is worthless, faces frequent physical attacks from which she cannot escape, has no money to leave, and all her efforts to cope are thwarted. Ultimately she stops trying to change her situation or leave it. She lives with chronic depression. Seligman would say she had developed learned helplessness.

In summary, it is clear that the causes of mood disorders can be attributed to a variety of biological, psychological, and social factors that combine in complex ways to precipitate depression or bipolar disorder. Genetic and psychological vulnerabilities may predispose the individual to mood problems when combined with a precipitating environmental event. The interactions are intriguing, and researchers are only beginning to understand how these factors interrelate to produce a specific disorder.

TREATMENT OF MOOD DISORDERS

Depression may be one of the most treatable of all psychiatric disorders. Regrettably, it goes undiagnosed and untreated all too often by medical professionals and misunderstood by many of those affected by the disorder. Somatic, psychopharmacological, and psychological treatments have advanced dramatically in the past 40 years and have given relief to many who in the past would have suffered throughout their entire lives.

Since depression may manifest itself along a continuum from mild situational dysfunction to severe major depression with psychotic features, it follows that effective treatments will also vary. The most severe and debilitating mood disorders like major depression and bipolar disorder, both with clear genetic and biological roots, respond effectively to medication and other somatic interventions. Milder forms of depression that tend to involve more transient, environmental stressors can be treated very effectively with psychological therapies. However, most outcome research comparing groups of depressed patients treated with medication only, those treated with cognitive psychotherapy only, and those treated with a combination of both approaches have found that improvement was most significant for those patients treated with a combination of treatments.

The primary form of somatic therapy for depression involves the administration of antidepressant medication. There are three major classes of drugs that are currently employed by medical professionals to treat depression: tricyclic anti-depressants, monoamine oxidase inhibitors and selective serotonergic uptake inhibitors. Tricyclic anti-depressants (e.g. Tofranil and Elavil) are an older class of drugs and are thought to work by blocking the reuptake of certain neurosynaptic transmitters like norepinephrine, ultimately making more of these chemical messengers available at the synapse, allowing continued stimulation along the brain circuit. Thus, the theory goes, once the normal balance of chemicals is restored by the medication, the depressive symptoms lift. Tricyclic anti-depressants often result in a number of uncomfortable side effects including constipation, dry mouth, blurred vision, weight gain and sexual dysfunction, but are quite effective in 50–60% of patients in addressing the depressive symptoms. However, the greatest problem with these drugs involves the potential toxic effects on cardiac functioning and the very significant possibilities of a lethal overdose in suicidal patients.

MAO Inhibitors (Parnate) work by blocking the enzyme monoamine oxidase that breaks down transmitters including serotonin and norepinephrine, allowing those chemical messengers to be more available at the synapse, leading to what the theory refers to as down-regulation or desensitization at the synapse. These drugs have also demonstrated their effectiveness, but are used infrequently because serious hypertensive crises result when the patient eats or drinks foods like cheese or red wine that contain tryamine.

The newest class of drugs, called Serotonergic Selective Reuptake Inhibitors, work by blocking the reabsorbtion or "reuptake" of serotonin at the synapse, temporarily making it more available at the receptor site. By affecting the serotonin brain pathways more specifically, this class of drugs results in fewer of the uncomfortable and dangerous side effects of earlier anti-depressants, although their effectiveness is comparable. SSRI's including Prozac, Zoloft and Paxil nevertheless have their own side effects, including sexual dysfunction, agitation, weight gain and insomnia.

Another antidepressant drug called lithium is more commonly associated with the treatment of the manic episode of bipolar disorders and is part of the class of drugs called *mood stabilizers*. While the mechanism of action is unclear, lithium works by stabilizing mood and preventing the patient from "cycling" from one mood state to another. Researchers suspect that it limits the availability of transmitters including dopamine and norepinephrine and has effects on neurohormones in the endocrine system. While a significant number of patients respond well to this drug, it is prescribed cautiously since it can be very toxic unless regulated carefully. Other mood stabilizing drugs, including Depakote and Trileptal, are classed as anticonvulsants and are effective for many patients who do not benefit from lithium. Box 3.4 lists these and other commonly used medications for depression.

For those severe mood disordered patients whose response to medication has been poor, electroconvulsive therapy may be the treatment of choice. Research indicates that, while it has become associated with discredited treatments like psychosurgery and insulin shock therapy so often perpetrated on patients in the past, ECT has a 90% effectiveness rate with medication resistant patients. Patients receive anesthesia and feel no discomfort as an electric shock is delivered to the brain, producing a convulsion. Typically, the patient will undergo a series of treatments over several weeks and then be placed on medication once again to prevent relapse. The mechanism of action is unknown and the side effects profile is limited to some short-term memory loss and confusion, both of which are generally transient.

It has been noted by some researchers that a combination of drug treatment and psychotherapy has been shown to be most effective in treating mood disorders, especially depression. Drug therapy is more likely to effect symptomatic changes more quickly, while psychosocial interventions provide the patient more insight and coping skills to address problems around their ongoing functioning.

Several psychological approaches are utilized in the treatment of depression. Psychodynamic approaches focus on exploring childhood developmental experiences, many of which may be unconscious, which arouse feelings of loss, guilt, and, ultimately, depressive symptoms. Perhaps among the most researched and popular approaches today are cognitive therapy and interpersonal psychotherapy. Cognitive therapy builds on the notion that negative thinking, unrealistic and often irrational appraisals of themselves, the world and the future result in depression. Therapists then help the patient to identify their overgeneralizations and black and white thinking, their negative assumptions and beliefs that are unsupported with reality-based information and to substitute more rational beliefs. Patients learn how their feelings and behavior are determined in large measure by their thinking and that, by challenging their irrational beliefs, they can experience a reduction in their depression.

Interpersonal psychotherapy emphasizes the role of interpersonal relations in triggering mood problems. Therapists assist patients in resolving disputes like marital problems, resolving issues of loss of loved ones, in developing new relationships, and in developing effective social skills that insure effective interpersonal relationships.

While potentially all patients can benefit from individual or group psychotherapy in treating their mood disorders, clinicians and researchers generally emphasize the biological underpinnings of bipolar illness and focus primarily on medication management to treat the disorder. Psychological interventions with bipolar patients tend to focus on patient and family education about the illness, counseling to insure medication compliance and family treatment of the often destructive consequences of a manic episode. Marital, financial and interpersonal fallout from a manic episode are often devastating after a patient, hindered by extremely poor judgment, engages in inappropriate sexual, gambling, financial, and often anti-social behavior. Without appropriate psychosocial intervention, the risk of relapse in the bipolar patient is very high.

MOOD DISORDERS AND CHILDREN

Mood disorders do occur in childhood, but less frequently than in adults. Adolescents, however, show increasing rates of depression and bipolar disorder. Accurate diagnosis is important here to insure that these children and adolescents receive appropriate treatment rather than punishment through the juvenile justice system.

The most common of the mood disorders in children are those that incorporate some of the signs and symptoms of depression. This includes a chronic sad mood that is diagnosed as Dysthymic Disorder if it lasts more than 1 year, and a Major Depressive Disorder (MDD) with episodes of depression that last for several months at a time. As children often display irritability and even hostility instead of a continuous sad mood, it is more difficult to diagnose MDD in children than it is in adults. However, like adults, the symptoms get more intense and last longer each time there is a new episode of depression.

Children, especially adolescents have ups and downs as part of their development, but mania in Bipolar Disorder is very different. There is a frenetic quality to manic behavior where the behavior in question seems to keep escalating beyond what is considered appropriate. The average of onset of Bipolar Disorder in children is around age 10, but it has been diagnosed in children as young as 2 years old. Many of the same signs and symptoms seen in adults, such as the pressured rapid speech, are also seen in children going through the manic phase. Sometimes the manic phase is confused with Attention Deficit/Hyperactivity Disorder or Post Traumatic Stress Disorder, and it is not unusual to find these three disorders in the same person, especially after experiencing a trauma.

Anti-depressants, mood stabilizers, and atypical anti-psychotic medications may be prescribed to treat children who have depression, mania and wide mood swings, but it is often difficult to motivate them or their parents to continue to take the medications. Teenagers, like adults, may enjoy the "highs" and resist giving them up despite the pressures to conform. Psychotherapy, even without medication, has also been proven to be effective in stabilizing children's moods.

SUICIDE

Probably the most devastating consequence of a mood disorder is suicide. Research has indicated that approximately 60% of suicides are associated with an existing mood disorder, although many individuals without that diagnosis complete suicide. First Responders will have the opportunity to deal with this very serious problem more often, perhaps, than any other psychological crisis or disorder.

Successful suicide, a national problem with over 30,000 people completing suicide each year, is the eighth leading cause of death in the United States. Researchers claim unreported suicides to be significantly higher. Law enforcement and emergency personnel deal with car accidents and occupational deaths each day that may very well be actual suicides. In recent years, there has been an alarming increase in adolescent suicides that today are the third leading cause of death among teenagers, behind motor vehicle accidents and homicides.

According to the 2006 report of the National Institute of Mental Health, the highest suicide rates in the United States are found in white men over the age of 85. Men have a completed suicide rate that is four times greater than women, although women attempt suicide two to three times as often as men. The difference is due in large part to the fact that men choose more lethal methods, including guns and hanging, while women are more likely to overdose on pills or slash their wrists, methods that have the possibility of being "undone." Additionally, given the fact that women are twice as likely to develop depression, the odds are greater that suicide might be an outcome. While there are no absolute predictors of suicide, several risk factors involving clinical, historical, and demographic factors will alert the First Responder to those individuals most in need of intervention and treatment. The table below summarizes these key factors (Box 6.1).

Suicide in Youth

Suicide is the third leading cause of death in adolescents, with only accidents and homicides being higher, according to the U.S. Bureau of Statistics. Much like the data for adults, boys are most likely to use guns and hanging as the methods to die, while girls are more likely to intentionally ingest toxic substances than use a gun. In a survey of U.S. high school students, close to one-fifth (20%) admitted having suicidal thoughts, while almost 10% attempted suicide. Only 2.6% of those actually received medical attention, and less than one in one hundred were successful (0.008%). The few studies of children who are successful at committing suicide suggest that both depression that has been noted and a family history of suicide are factors that may predispose a child to killing him or herself. Interestingly, in a few studies of depressed youth who were successful in committing suicide, in the 25% of them

BOX 6.1	Clinical/Psychological
Risk Factors for Suicide	Mood disorders
	Feelings of hopelessness
Historical/Demographic	Substance abuse/dependence
History of prior suicide attempt(s)	Chronic pain/terminal illness
Family history of suicide	Loss (health, relationship, support)
Family history of physical/sexual abuse	Impulsive/angry behavior
Males in general	Well-conceived suicide plan
Single, divorced, separated, widowed	Accessibility to lethal method
Teenagers and elderly	Legal problems/incarceration
Caucasians and Native Americans	Humiliating life event (arrest)
Gays, lesbians and bisexuals	
Police officers, dentists, physicians	
Unemployed	

who were prescribed medication for their depression, none had taken it at the time of their death since it was not found in autopsy. Most important is the information that it is not uncommon for adolescents to have suicidal ideation that they are particularly adept at covering up unless directly asked about it.

Dealing with Suicide

Faced with a person threatening suicide or one who has been identified as having suicidal thoughts or manifesting self-destructive suicidal gestures (self-mutilation, frequent overdosing), First Responders will have a crucial role. Encouraging subjects to talk about their frustrations, hopelessness, or anger will communicate a willingness to reach out to them when so often the suicidal individual feels cut off from others and socially isolated. Responding to the core feeling of hopelessness by offering the opportunity to address the problem with assistance from others will at the very least provide the subjects with the opportunity to reconsider their decision, particularly when it results from an impulsive, stress related reaction. Ultimately, if the First Responder decides that the individuals pose an imminent danger to themselves as a result of mental illness, it will be their responsibility to consider "arresting" the subject and transporting them to a facility for psychiatric evaluation and stabilization.

One of the most challenging situations law enforcement officers will face involves the decision to fire their weapon when confronted with a subject threatening them with a lethal weapon. Administrative reviews of shootings typically attempt to assess whether an appropriate level of force was used to deal with the shooter. When the subject has encouraged or challenged the police officer to employ deadly force, this after the fact assessment becomes even more complex. In many of these cases, the officer may have encountered a suicidal and/or mentally ill person who has chosen "suicide by cop." Many cases are on record of police firing on individuals who are threatening with fire arms that turn out, upon investigation, to be unloaded weapons, toy guns, or starter pistols. Often suicidal motivation is difficult or impossible to establish, while some cases are rather clear-cut. Reviews of shootings have revealed chronic histories of mental illness or suicidal behavior that clearly raise the likelihood of "suicide by cop." In the best of situations, the subjects may try to verbally provoke the officer to kill them, thereby revealing their true motivation and, in so doing, they increase the possibility of a successful intervention, avoidance of harm, and eventual treatment.

Why would a suicidal person choose to die in this way? We may speculate that the individual has chosen to die, but refuses to kill him- or herself out of fear of the unknown, refusal to take personal responsibility for his or her death, or perhaps an unwillingness to "pull the trigger." Underlying much suicidal behavior are anger and rage. By confronting police with threats of attack or invitations to be killed, this rage is discharged on the police as well as indirectly turned on themselves.

The problem of "suicide by cop" is undoubtedly one of significance that has an estimated involvement in up to 40% of police shootings. The phenomenon impacts on the civilian community's concerns over the inappropriate use of deadly force, on the overwhelming psychological stress on officers themselves, and on the possibility that suggesting the presence of suicidal motivation in a subject of a police shooting may look as if the officer is avoiding responsibility for poor judgment. Clearly, First Responders have a responsibility to be aware of the most effective ways to handle such crisis situations, to be knowledgeable about suicidal motivation and indicators of suicidal lethality, and to seek to develop procedures for psychological autopsies that will give us insight into the minds of victims of "suicide by cop."

SUGGESTED READINGS

Beck, A. T. (1987). *Cognitive therapy of depression*. New York: Guilford Press.
Beckham, E. E. & Leber, W. R. (Eds.). (1995). *Handbook of depression*. New York: Guilford.
Beiling, P. J. & Antony, M. M. (2003). *Ending the depression cycle: A step-by-step guide for preventing relapse*. New Harbinger Publications.
Burns, D. D. (1989). *The feeling good handbook*. New York: Plume.
Castle, L. R. (2002). *Bi-polar disorder demystified*. New York: Marlowe and Company.
Cicchetti, D. & Toth, S. (Eds.). (1992). *Developmental perspectives on depression*. Rochester New York: University of Rochester Press.
Craig, K. D. & Dobson, K. S. (Eds.). (1995). *Anxiety and depression in adults and children*. Thousand Oaks, CA: Sage Publications.
Den Boer, J. A. & Sitsen, A. (Eds.). (1994). *Handbook of depression and anxiety*. New York: Marcel Dekker.

Faedda, G., Tondo, L., & Ross, J. (1993). *Seasonal mood disorders: Patterns of seasonal recurrence in mania and depression.* New York: New Harbinger.

Fristad, M. A. & Goldberg, Arnold, J. S. (2004). *Raising a moody child: How to cope with depression and bi-polar disorder.* New York: Gulford Press.

Goodwin, F. K. & Jamison, K. R. (1990). *Manic-depressive illness.* New York: Oxford University Press.

Ingram, R. E., Miranda, J., & Segal, Z. V. (1998). *Cognitive vulnerability to depression.* New York: Guilford Press.

Leahy, R. L. & Johnson, S. L. (Eds.). (2005). *Psychological treatment of bi-polar disorder.* New York: Guilford Press.

Maj, M., Akiskal, H. S., & Lopez-Ibar, J. J. (2002). *Bi-polar disorder.* New York: John Wiley and Sons.

Paykel, E. S. (Ed.). (1992). *Handbook of affective disorders.* New York: Guilford Press.

Seligman, M. E. P. (2002). *Authentic happiness: Using the new positive psychology to realize your potential for lasting fulfillment.* New York: Free Press/Simon and Schuster.

Shneidman, E. S., Farberow, N. L., and Litman, R. E. (Eds.). (1970). *The psychology of suicide.* New York: Science House.

Thayer, R. E. (1996). *The origin of everyday moods.* New York: Oxford University Press.

Torrey, E. F. & Knable, M. B. (2005). *Surviving manic depression.* New York: Basic Books.

CHAPTER 7

The Anxiety, Somatoform and Dissociative Disorders

ANXIETY DISORDERS

The experience of anxiety and fear is a common one for personnel involved in dangerous, high risk situations with life and death consequences. In fact, First Responders benefit from the increased autonomic nervous system response that accompanies anxiety and fear and that mobilizes their resources to flee from a dangerous scene or remain and aggressively confront it. In the early 1900s, researcher Walter Cannon described this reaction to danger as the "fight or flight response." Some degree of anxiety facilitates performance in many areas. It helps to focus our attention, to anticipate possible negative consequences of our behavior, and generally to keep us "up" to face difficult emergency situations, perform well on tests or even respond thoughtfully to an attorney's aggressive cross examination. This chapter, however, will focus primarily on anxiety that has reached exaggerated and self defeating levels that impair performance, cause significant impairment in functioning, and reach the threshold for a formal psychiatric disorder. Additionally, we will touch briefly on those psychological disorders in which the individuals suffer from concern over physical symptoms or a belief that they have a disease for which no identifiable medical basis can be found. These disorders are labeled Somatoform disorders. Emergency medical personnel may occasionally deal with such patients.

Dimensions of Anxiety

In differentiating anxiety from a fear reaction, many experts assert that anxiety is related to worry about future events that are frequently uncontrollable, whereas fear is our immediate reaction to current danger. We will not address the possible theoretical differences between these constructs, but will focus only on anxiety as a negative mood state that manifests itself in at least four domains including somatic, cognitive, motor, and affective.

87

BOX 7.1

Can You Diagnose Which Anxiety Disorder?

Can you figure out which anxiety disorder this law enforcement officer, Detective Miller, has upon being required to testify in a court hearing? Remember, what diagnosis will be given will depend upon **what** he fears, **why** it is feared, and **how** he expresses his fear.

Scenario One: Detective Miller fears being unable to escape from the courtroom **(what)** when he begins to testify **(why)**. He starts to experience a panic attack that is expressed in physiological reactions including heart palpitations, dizziness, hyperventilation, and fear of losing control **(how)**.

Scenario Two: Detective Miller is afraid of scrutiny by others in court **(what)** and the possibility of acting in a way that would be embarrassing **(why)** and this is expressed by the avoidance of the situation **(how)**.

Scenario Three: Detective Miller does not want to testify in court **(what)** because

he is concerned about contamination from dirt that he would come in contact with on the witness stand or on the courtroom doorknobs **(why)**. He would manifest cognitive symptoms of obsessions about contamination and compulsive cleaning rituals and he would ruminate about it **(how)**.

Scenario Four: Detective Miller does not want to testify in court **(what)** because at one time he was traumatized by a prisoner who threatened his life when he took him hostage **(why)**. He still has nightmares, feelings of apathy and emotional numbness, feels nervous and jumpy at times, and cannot recall some of the event at times **(how)**.

Answers:

Scenario one—Panic Disorder with Agoraphobia
Scenario two—Social Phobia
Scenario three—Obsessive Compulsive Disorder
Scenario four—Post Traumatic Stress Disorder

Anyone who has experienced severe anxiety may recall excessive sweating, feelings of weakness, dry mouth, flushing, dizziness, heart palpitations, hyperventilation, and headaches or gastrointestinal distress that represent the somatic domain. Cognitive symptoms often include worry, feelings of dread or impending disaster, vague fears of dying or even "going crazy." Additionally, high levels of anxiety will impair concentration rather than enhance it, and cause extreme distractibility. Motor impairments include tremulousness, tics, shaking, jumpiness, pacing, over reactivity to minor stimuli, and hypervigilance. Finally, affective or emotional symptoms may include feelings of tenseness, panicky feelings, dysphoria, and irritability. Obviously, these domains overlap, but as we will see, specific anxiety disorders may be characterized primarily by symptoms from one particular domain or another.

In order to understand some of the similarities and differences among the major anxiety disorders, the reader can ask three important questions: (1) What is feared?; (2) Why is it feared?; and (3) How is it feared? See Box 7.1 for answers to these questions.

The reader will notice that the object of fear and anxiety is the same in this case (courtroom), but the basis for the fear and the symptoms associated with it are very different. The anxiety symptoms all represent one of the four domains described earlier.

Panic Disorder with and without Agoraphobia

The officer in the example feared having a panic attack when in the courtroom (Table 7.1). A panic attack is described in *DSM-IV-TR* as a discrete period of intense fear or discomfort lasting several minutes and manifested by a variety of physiological and cognitive symptoms such as palpitations, sweating, shaking, breathing difficulties, fear of losing control or going crazy, tingling in the extremities, and fear of dying. The panic attack is one of the most frightening forms of anxiety and can occur in several different anxiety disorders including the phobias, as well as panic disorder with and without agoraphobia. When panic attacks occur unexpectedly and recurrently, cause individuals significant concern over having more attacks and/or cause them to change their behavior in anticipation of a panic attack, we make the diagnosis of *Panic Disorder*.

Panic Disorder may come on acutely and at times even wake individuals up from a sound sleep. Typically, the first time individuals experience an episode, they fear they are having a coronary and will decide to go to an emergency room. After proper evaluation they will be treated for anxiety, and frequently they will be referred to a mental health professional. The experience of panic attacks can be perceived as so distressing and life threatening that individuals begin fearing that they will experience the attack in a situation in which no help is available and from which escape would be impossible or at least embarrassing. Often patients will have panic attacks when driving their cars in heavy traffic, on bridges, in tunnels, or when shopping in malls. Many will decide to avoid those situations and begin to restrict their travel, some even confining themselves to their home where they feel most safe. When individuals with Panic Disorder begin this type of avoidance, we make the diagnosis of *Panic Disorder with Agoraphobia*. While the term has the literal meaning of "fear of the marketplace," in effect, the individual really fears having a panic attack in situations from which

Table 7.1. Cardinal Signs and Symptoms: Panic Attack

- Pounding heart
- Sweating
- Tremulousness
- Breathing difficulties
- Feeling of choking
- Chest discomfort
- GI distress
- Dizziness
- Feelings of unreality
- Fear of going crazy or dying
- Numbness/pins and needles
- Chills or hot flashes

they could not escape or receive help. Consequently, agoraphobia really is the "fear of fear." Sometimes patients will have no history of panic attacks, but continue to avoid situations in which they experience some anxiety or anticipate having attacks. In that case we would diagnose Agoraphobia without History of Panic Attacks.

Panic Disorder with and without Agoraphobia is quite prevalent in the population with around 3% of the population experiencing an episode at some point in their lives. Approximately 6 million American adults ages 18 and older have Panic Disorder in a given year. Women are twice as likely to suffer from Panic Disorder as men. Average age of onset is around 25 years old.

Understanding the causes of Panic Disorder requires an integration of multiple sources of influence including biological vulnerability, psychological predisposition, and stress that combine to bring about the disorder. As in other disorders we have discussed, genetic factors may play an important role in creating the threshold for experiencing panic when under stress. The disorder seems to run in families. Some individuals also learn to view the world as dangerous and will perceive situations as frightening and respond with panic attacks when faced with a variety of stressors. Many authorities believe that panic attacks become conditioned to physiological stress reactions like increased heart rate or even certain experiences like exercise or angry feelings that trigger the panic reaction. Patients begin to associate these feelings or situations with panic and interpret their feelings as a signal that an attack is imminent. The expectation begins to snowball, causing more anxiety and confirmation of their catastrophic belief until they have a full blown panic attack. Other experts focus on psychological conflicts around separation anxiety in childhood and frustrated dependency conflicts as the cause of panic disorder. They assert that the loss of dependent supports trigger panic reactions when individuals face crises like divorce, death of loved ones, or loss of a job.

Treatment for Panic Disorder with and without Agoraphobia typically involves some combination of medication and psychotherapy. Both SSRI's and benzodiazepines have shown their effectiveness for this problem, and patients tend to do quite well as long as they maintain the medication regimen. However, outcome research consistently indicates that psychological interventions, especially exposure to the feared situations, are quite effective, allow the individual to discover that their fears are unfounded, and that they can master their panic through skills like diaphragmatic breathing and relaxation training. Additionally, cognitive therapy teaches patients to view their situations more realistically and avoid misinterpreting somatic cues that have been the stimuli for anxiety and panic.

Generalized Anxiety Disorder

Unlike the acute and dramatic nature of Panic Disorder that focuses primarily on autonomic nervous system arousal, *Generalized Anxiety Disorder* (GAD) presents as chronic and excessive worry over a litany of

Table 7.2. Cardinal Signs and Symptoms: Generalized Anxiety Disorder

- Extreme worry and anxiety over many issues
- Inability to control the worry
- Feelings of restlessness
- Easily fatigued
- Difficulty concentrating
- Irritability
- Muscle tension
- Sleep problems

events, activities, or situations in the patient's life (Table 7.2). The worrying is usually unproductive, and the individual feels little or no control over shutting off the worry. Individuals experience their anxiety as restlessness, fatigue, muscle tension or irritability and typically suffer from sleep difficulty. The anxiety manifested in GAD tends to be more anticipatory of future threat than immediate threat experienced in Panic Disorder.

GAD is quite common in the population and the lifetime prevalence has been reported as high as 6% in the United States. The disorder tends to develop rather insidiously and is generally chronic, affecting many elderly persons. It shares a high co-morbidity with Major Depression where up to 40% of patients with GAD also suffer from serious depression.

A combination of biological and psychological vulnerabilities seems to predispose individuals to GAD. Researchers and clinicians recognize that in combination with a genetic diathesis as a biological foundation, individuals may develop beliefs early in life that their world is uncontrollable and dangerous, and these beliefs demand that they be highly vigilant and on guard against potential threats. Worrying results from this vigilance and represents the cardinal symptom of GAD.

Treatment for GAD generally focuses on use of medications to manage the patient's anxiety. Benzodiazepines like Valium, Ativan and Xanax are quite effective, although they bring with them the risk of dependence when used for long periods of time. Anti-depressants including Paxil, Zoloft, and Effexor are also used and avoid the risk of dependence. Overdose with the benzodiazepines can be more dangerous than with the SSRI's and so are more likely to be prescribed for impulsive or suicidal individuals. Psychological interventions, including relaxation training and cognitive-behavioral treatment, are often employed and may be more effective in the long term, but most individuals with the disorder will often require medication to allay their discomfort and allow them to cope with their chronic anxiety and worry.

Specific Phobia

Many of us can describe certain situations or objects that cause us enough anxiety and discomfort that we choose to avoid rather than face

Table 7.3. Cardinal Signs and Symptoms: Specific Phobia

- Excessive or unreasonable fear of a specific object or situation
- Exposure to object causes a panic attack
- Individual recognizes fear is unreasonable
- Object is avoided or tolerated with distress

them. High places, thunderstorms, or snakes have in common the tendency to cause many individuals to feel this discomfort and to motivate them to stay away. Most of us can relate to one or more of these concerns, but generally find a way to deal with them without much effort or disruption in our lives. However, when the exposure to such situations or objects causes individuals to experience a debilitating panic attack and requires them to make major accommodations in their lives that impair their overall functioning, the reaction rises to the level of a *Specific Phobia* (Table 7.3).

DSM-IV-TR describes a specific phobia as a marked fear of a specific object or situation that is excessive and unreasonable, and invariably provokes anxiety in the form of a panic attack. While individuals will recognize and admit that their fear is irrational, they will not be able to control their reaction and will either avoid the situation/object altogether or experience much discomfort in its presence. The diagnostic manual divides the Specific Phobia into several subtypes including animal, natural environment (water), blood injection-injury, situational (fear of flying, enclosed places) and other (choking, clowns).

Specific Phobia is the second most common anxiety disorder with a lifetime prevalence of up to about 11%. Women are significantly more likely than men to develop the disorder. Some of the more common phobias are heights, insects, illness, and storms. Unlike GAD and Panic Disorder, patients diagnosed with Specific Phobias do not experience general autonomic arousal except when they are exposed to the actual situation. Rather, they are able to displace their anxiety onto a specific situation or object and experience no discomfort as long as they can avoid them.

As with many other psychological disorders, the etiology of Specific Phobias is not clear-cut. Many research studies suggest that phobias are learned based on past negative experience with an object or situation, through observing another person react with fear to the situation or even through experiencing a panic attack in the presence of the object. In this latter way, the neutral object or situation has been conditioned to anxiety and will elicit a fear reaction whenever the individual encounters it. Other research, however, has found that up to 27% of phobics surveyed had no recollection of the origin of their problem. Research has also suggested a biological or genetic predisposition for developing the problem, in particular for the blood/injection-injury type phobia. One author found 64% of the 25 patients interviewed had at least one first degree biological relative with a blood phobia. In contrast

BOX 7.2	He deals with this by refusing to carry a
Phobia	weapon and by requesting administrative
An officer who has ongoing conflict with his estranged wife and about whom he feels overwhelming anger and rage, may develop a Specific Phobia of weapons.	duty. Unconsciously the phobia symbolizes his murderous impulses and by avoiding weapons he protects himself from acting on those impulses.

to more behaviorally oriented researchers, psychodynamic clinicians may conceptualize phobias as symbols of unconscious conflict. By avoiding the feared object or situation, the individual avoids dealing with the underlying intrapsychic conflict that would arouse overwhelming anxiety and psychological pain. See Box 7.2 for a case example.

Behavioral treatment for Specific Phobias commonly centers on exposing the patient to the feared object or situation, but doing so in a very gradual way. The patient tolerates small steps in getting closer and closer to the phobic object, tolerating increasing amounts of anxiety until he/she is able to face the situation rather than avoid it. Dynamic therapists might explore the patient's current life situation and past history looking for underlying conflicts, trauma, or feelings that have been unconsciously represented by the phobia, and then helping the patient become aware of and deal more effectively with the problem.

Social Phobia

Many individuals avoid performance situations where they will be faced with potential evaluation or scrutiny by others. We all know people who fear public speaking and avoid at all costs meetings, classes or social gatherings where they must speak in front of others. Many children as well as adults are described as "shy" and struggle throughout their lives to deal with social situations in which they feel uncomfortable and avoid interacting with others in group situations. When "shyness" rises to the level of absolute avoidance of those social situations or to panic attacks when forced to enter them, we begin considering the diagnosis of *Social Phobia* and the potential need for treatment. Perhaps less common, but equally uncomfortable for some, are situations involving signing one's name in front of others, acting in a play or performing professionally as musicians or artists. A relatively common social phobia for men involves urinating in a public restroom, sometimes referred to as "shy bladder." In all these cases, individuals fear evaluation or scrutiny by others and believe that they will be judged negatively. They typically either avoid the situation or, when unable to escape, experience a panic attack or very debilitating anxiety that often will impair their daily functioning.

Social phobia is the most common anxiety disorder with around 13% of the general population suffering from it. Usually the disorder begins in early adolescence and is likely to have its origins in an inherited inhibited temperament that may be reinforced by environmental events during which individuals learn that social evaluation is dangerous or that they are vulnerable to attacks from others in social situations. Psychotherapy using cognitive-behavioral techniques involving the challenging of irrational beliefs about social situations and gradual exposure to the feared situations has proven helpful in addressing the problem. For many individuals, psychotropic medication is employed in reducing their debilitating anxiety, allowing them not only to feel better psychologically in social environments, but also to perform more competently. Specific types of medications that reduce those physical symptoms of anxiety like heart palpitations, dry mouth and tremulousness that impair performance are often prescribed, even though the individual may continue to feel uncomfortable psychologically.

Separation Anxiety Disorder

Separation Anxiety Disorder is diagnosed in 4% of all children, more commonly in younger children and less commonly as they reach adolescence. The mean age of onset is 7.5 years old, but many young children exhibit separation anxiety especially when separated from a parent, usually their mother, such as when they enter school for the first time. This disorder is associated with a myriad of fears in the young child. Although it is not considered a serious disorder, the anxiety can manifest itself in many different ways as children grow up. Children under the age of eight years old center their anxiety around the safety of their parents and school refusal. Typically, the intervention for these children is to help them face their fears and learn that it will not be devastating when they are not with a parent.

Children who are ages nine to twelve years old typically have excessive distress at the time of any separation. Adolescents ages 12 to 16 may have limited independent activities and a renewal of their school refusal that may have been seen when they were younger. They may also have somatic symptoms associated with their anxiety.

Obsessive-Compulsive Disorder

At one time or the other we all struggle with getting things "off our mind." Preoccupation with a problem at home or work that we cannot shake, a persistent image that might be disquieting, or even a song that reverberates in our head to the point of annoyance are relatively common experiences. We also may engage in certain ritualistic behavior that we feel compelled to perform. Superstitious behavior falls into this category. "Knocking on wood," avoiding walking under ladders, or even following a very prescribed order for dressing in the morning are all geared to help us feel more comfortable in our world. Even though they are not realistically useful, we find ourselves engaging in them in order to prevent something "bad" from happening. Generally, these thoughts and behaviors are not disruptive and cause little if any emotional discomfort. However, individuals with *Obsessive-Compulsive Disorder* (OCD) experience

Table 7.4. Cardinal Signs and Symptoms: Obessive-Compulsive Disorder

- Recurrent thoughts, images or impulses that are intrusive, inappropriate and causes distress
- Person tries to ignore or neutralize them with other thoughts or behavior
- Person recognizes that thoughts are product of their own mind
- Repetitive behaviors that person is driven to perform like counting or handwashing
- The behaviors are ways to reduce distress or some feared event but are not realistic
- These obsession and compulsions impair a person's daily functioning

exaggerated forms of these thoughts and behaviors that result in overwhelming anxiety and dramatically impaired daily functioning (Table 7.4).

OCD is characterized by either obsessions or compulsions that consume significant amounts of time in the person's life and that the individual recognizes are unreasonable and excessive. *Obsessions* are recurrent thoughts, images or ideas that the individuals experience as intrusive and persistent, but recognizes that they are the product of their own minds and not imposed from without. Common obsessions include thoughts of contamination, hostility, and sexual imagery that the person tries to resist or eliminate by thinking of another thought or engaging in some magical behavior. A fear of stabbing your child in the eye, the idea that your house will burn down, or feeling the impulse to jump out in front of traffic are obsessive ideas that cause the person overwhelming anxiety that often can be eliminated only by engaging in a compulsive act.

Compulsions involve repetitive, ritualized behaviors that the individual must perform in order to prevent some catastrophic event or neutralize an obsessive idea or impulse. One of the defining characteristics of compulsions is their magical nature since they are not realistically connected to the idea or impulse they are designed to eliminate. Common compulsions involve cleaning, checking and ordering. A patient presented to a psychologist complaining that his hands were severely chapped after washing his hands 300 times a day to prevent contamination with HIV. Another woman spent hours each night before bedtime checking that each appliance in her home was unplugged, fearing that her house would burn down.

The lifetime prevalence of OCD is about 2.5%. Onset ranges from early adolescence to mid-20s with a pattern of chronic impairment once the disorder develops. Like several of the other disorders that have been described, OCD involves a biological diathesis or predisposition that interacts with psychological stress, disruptive family environments, and learned magical behaviors conditioned to eliminate anxiety. One research study of identical twins found that if one co-twin developed OCD, there was a 57% chance that the other twin would also develop the disorder.

Scientists have found that SSRI's designed to limit the reuptake of the neurosynaptic transmitter serotonin have a positive effect on minimizing the symptoms of OCD. Psychological treatments involve behavioral techniques including thought stopping (yelling "stop" when experiencing an obsession) and response prevention where patients are prevented from engaging in a compulsive behavior when gradually exposed to the obsession or feared situation. Typically, these procedures work best in a fairly restrictive environment like a hospital where the patient cannot easily avoid facing the frightening situation. While psychological and medical treatment have reduced the symptoms of OCD at times to manageable levels, the disorder remains very difficult to treat effectively.

Law enforcement personnel and other First Responders are likely to be familiar with several disorders that seem to share some commonalities with OCD, particularly the compulsive symptoms. Kleptomania, Pyromania, Pathological Gambling, Intermittent Explosive Disorder all appear at first glance to have a compulsive quality, but are in fact classified in the DSM, not as OCD, but as Impulse Control Disorders. Stalking behavior can be added to this list since it often combines obsessional and compulsive components. Each of these disorders will be described below.

Kleptomania involves a rather persistent and recurring impulse to steal things that have no real value and for which the individual has no use. The motivation to steal is apparently unconscious and the individual appears to respond to feelings of tension followed by pleasure or relief while the item is being stolen. While it is typical that the person will not steal when in plain sight of the police, perpetrators generally do not premeditate the crime, consider the potential consequences, or involve accomplices. Generally, these individuals understand that their behavior is wrong and experience guilt after the act. This reaction is in sharp distinction to the criminal or sociopath who steals for profit and feels no guilt or the delinquent adolescent who shoplifts for personal gain, to act on a dare or as a way to rebel against authority. This disorder is very rare and tends to be more common in women.

Pyromania involves the irresistible impulse to set fires. Just as most shoplifters are not kleptomaniacs, most arsonists are not pyromaniacs. The latter group experience rising tension before they act and feelings of tension release or pleasure as they witness the fire, usually remaining at the scene to observe the act. Many pyromaniacs are fascinated by fire equipment and the technology associated with it. This disorder is also very rare in the population. See Box 7.3 for a case example.

Pathological gambling has been increasing over the years with the increasing availability of gambling venues. Recent estimates indicate that 3 and 5% of adults are affected. Pathological gambling involves the self defeating preoccupation with gambling that leads to inability to stop despite severe consequences, lying to family and friends, and loss of

A delivery person for a major express company was arrested for setting fires in abandoned stores along the route that he delivered packages. He admitted being responsible for many small fires and several fires that went out of control and burned down entire blocks of houses and stores over a three year period. The firefighters recognized him as one of the onlookers who had been at several of the major fires. Although noticed, he did not seem out of the ordinary, and in fact, blended in with others from the neighborhood who came to watch the firefighters. During the initial interview with the police, he mentioned that he had enjoyed watching fires ever since he was a child when his mother started a fire in their home by falling asleep smoking a cigarette.

important relationships as well as illegal acts including forgery, theft, and embezzlement to support the habit. It shares the same inability to resist the impulse as the other disorders discussed above.

Intermittent explosive disorder is characterized by abrupt episodes of destructive or assaultive acts that are dramatically out of proportion to the precipitant. Law enforcement personnel deal with aggression and violence daily, but typically the aggression they confront is secondary to anti-social behavior, delinquency and, very often, substance intoxication, not intermittent explosive disorder. All other diagnoses must be eliminated before this rare disorder can be diagnosed. The etiology of IED has been associated with underlying neurobehavioral dysfunction including seizure disorders. A history of head injury is important to explore when considering this diagnosis. Often the primary treatments involve medication and biofeedback.

Stalking and erotomania are not formal diagnoses in the *DSM-IV-TR*, but they represent a problem that is very common. A recent study by the National Institute of Justice found that 8% of American women and 2% of American men will be stalked in their lifetimes. The vast majority of stalkers are men who typically are unable to let go of an intimate relationship that has ended. Many have been abusive in the relationship and have criminal histories for other offenses. They obsess about their "lost love" and define their personal value by maintaining the relationship. Not all stalkers have had any personal relationship or contact with their "victim." Some stalkers "believe" that they are destined to be with the victims and that they will succeed at convincing them if given enough time. This type of stalker tends to be a basically inadequate male with few social skills or history of intimate relationships whose belief about the victim's love may reach psychotic proportions. Psychologist Reid Malloy has studied the stalking behavior of those who perceive themselves in love with a famous person. A third type of stalker has been described as a "vengeful stalker." This applies to those who have become enraged at the victim for some perceived slight. This type of individual will often stalk old employers, politicians or co-workers to get retribution. Some batterers also fit this category. Law enforcement personnel should encourage victims to set firm boundaries with stalkers, refuse to compromise or appease them, and involve the authorities if the stalker persists.

PostTraumatic Stress Disorder

First Responders dedicate their lives to dealing with highly stressful situations that would overwhelm the average citizen (Table 7.5). Dealing with natural disasters, fires, and serious accidents in which victims are mutilated and killed, hostage situations and murders are among the traumatic events that police, paramedics, and firefighters face on a daily basis. Victims of these traumas who survive physically face the risk of developing an anxiety disorder called Post Traumatic Stress Disorder. In many cases these victims include the First Responders themselves. Some researchers have estimated that there is up to a 60% chance that emergency responders will develop PTSD symptoms at some point in their lives. According to the National Institute of Mental Health, approximately 7.7 million American adults age 18 and older, or about 3.5% of people in this age group in a given year, have PTSD.

In order to diagnose this disorder, *DSM-IV-TR* requires that individuals have been exposed to a traumatic event that could cause serious bodily harm or is life threatening, during which they felt intense fear and helplessness. First Responders will recognize that victims of such trauma may react in different ways at the time of the actual event. Some respond hysterically with evidence of agitation, screaming and crying, loss of bowel or bladder control, hyperactivity, and loss of emotional control. They may run back into a burning car or chase a rapist down the street. Others respond quite differently by becoming paralyzed, staring into space, fainting, or walking around aimlessly with eyes glazed over.

Table 7.5. Cardinal Signs and Symptoms: Posttraumatic Stress Disorder

- Person exposed to an event that involved actual or threatened death or injury to themselves or others
- Person responded with fear and helplessness
- Reexperiencing the event in recollections, dreams, flashbacks
- Intense distress when exposed to stimuli that symbolize the event
- Efforts to avoid any activities that aid in recalling event
- Inability to remember the trauma
- Loss of interest in activities
- Detachment from others
- Blunted affect
- Sleep disturbance
- Irritability and anger
- Concentration impairments
- Hypervigilence

BOX 7.4

PTSD

A sergeant, recently returned from Viet Nam, was brought to the emergency room in a state of agitation. He was combative with the MPs and medical staff, was not oriented to his situation and attempted to take the guard's weapon to apparently defend himself. He was not intoxicated and was sedated with medication until he became oriented and cooperative. The next day he was referred to the clinic psychologist for evaluation. At that time he was oriented in all spheres, very cooperative, docile and quite mild mannered. He had no recollection of his behavior the night before. A brief history of his experience in Viet Nam revealed an incident in which he led a platoon of infantrymen in the defense of a South Vietnamese village. They set up a perimeter around the area to prevent Viet Cong infiltrators from overrunning the small village. One evening the village was overrun and all of his men were killed but he—by the villagers themselves! His witnessing the annihilation of the men he was responsible for leading was too overwhelming to cope with and he ultimately developed PTSD. He added that a train whistle occurred during the original firefight. He remembered that a train whistle was the trigger for his decompensation the night before.

After the precipitating trauma, many individuals develop characteristic symptoms involving the re-experiencing of the event in the form of intrusive thoughts or images, nightmares, or flashbacks in which they relive the trauma as if it were actually re-occurring. Additionally, they may avoid any reminders of the trauma, have difficulty remembering the event, display a general numbing of emotional responsiveness, social withdrawal, and a sense of a foreshortened future. Finally, individuals with this diagnosis may have difficulty sleeping, display irritability, concentration problems, hypervigilance, and an exaggerated startle response. Some individuals will develop these symptoms very soon after the trauma, while others will manifest a delayed onset occurring six months or more after the precipitating event. A victim of domestic violence with a history of rape two years prior may develop full blown PTSD after having been verbally abused by her partner. This relatively minor event triggered a memory or image that re-ignited the original rape that had been "sealed over."

The soldier described in Box 7.4 experienced a flashback in the emergency room as he relived this traumatic episode. His mild manner and docile presentation are not unusual for victims of PTSD who may be dulled in emotional responsiveness. He described his trauma as if it were happening to someone else.

We may be surprised to learn that while many people have been exposed to a traumatic event in their lives, a relatively small number actually develop the symptoms of PTSD. Exposure to a traumatic situation in which the individual feels overwhelmed and helpless is necessary but not sufficient for the development of the disorder. One's genetic predisposition, family history of anxiety and other biological vulnerabilities, history of prior exposure to trauma, a learning history

involving the belief that events are uncontrollable, as well as the availability of a strong support system, all contribute to the actual expression
of the disorder. According to one study by Breslau and his colleagues in
1995, with the exception of rape, 75% of those exposed to trauma did
not have PTSD. Very close exposure to the traumatic situation is also a
necessary component. In Viet Nam, PTSD symptoms for men not
exposed to much combat reflected an incidence of about 7%.
Approximately 50 to 60% of men exposed to intense combat suffered
from the symptoms.

In treating the symptoms of PTSD, the conventional wisdom centers
on the use of a graded exposure to the original trauma in an effort to
desensitize the individual to the situation. In this way, the patient learns
to manage the anxiety and fear in small doses until the experience no
longer elicits the severe emotional reaction. SSRI's are also useful
adjuncts to treatment. There are several complications that arise in
treating the PTSD patient, including the co-morbidity of depression and
substance abuse. Estimates are that up to 50% of PTSD patients suffer
from depression, and 57% of males from alcoholism. These disorders
arising from the emotional pain of PTSD must also be treated.
Cognitive/behavior therapy, 12 step programs, as well as medications
designed for the treatment of anxiety and depression can be helpful.
Other programs including critical incident stress debriefing, group therapy and support groups will be discussed in another chapter focusing on
First Responders who struggle with stress related disorders as a result of
their chronic exposure to high stress environments.

SOMATOFORM DISORDERS

We have reviewed a number of disorders up to this point that involve
symptoms that revolve around thoughts, bizarre behaviors, anxiety,
depression and the like. In the case of somatoform disorders, patients
translate or "convert" their psychological pain, conflicts, fears, anxiety
or depression into physical representations that have no physiological or
organic basis. In other words, they experience and communicate their
psychological problems through their "soma" or body. Keep in mind
that patients with these diagnoses are not lying about their problems
and are not malingering for some personal gain, but truly "believe" that
they are ill or incapacitated. Upon physical examination, all tests are
negative or, in some cases, the patient's complaints or symptoms are
exaggerated and beyond what would be expected from their actual
physical problem. We know that somatic derivatives of psychological
problems are quite common in the general population, and it has been
estimated that up to 60% of all primary care physician visits have a
significant psychological basis. While these patients may not be suffering from a somatoform disorder, the statistic reveals the prevalence of

Table 7.6. Cardinal Signs and Symptoms: Somatization Disorder

- History of multiple physical complaints over several years and beginning before 30 years old
- Symptoms must occur across four systems:
  - Four pain symptoms
  - Two GI symptoms
  - One sexual symptom
  - One pseudoneurological symptom
- Cannot be fully explained by a medical/substance use condition or in excess of what would be predicted from an actual medical/substance use condition

psychological stress manifesting itself in symptoms like fatigue, headaches, GI distress, and chest pain that will signal a doctor visit to the primary care physician. This is further proof that the "mind and the body are connected."

Somatization Disorder

Patients with Somatization Disorder report a history of physical complaints that begin before the age of 30, occur over several years, cause significant impairment in their everyday functioning, yet have no firm medical basis (Table 7.6). These complaints must include a variety of symptoms covering four areas: at least four pain symptoms (i.e. in the head, extremities or during sexual intercourse); two gastrointestinal symptoms other than pain; one sexual symptom other than pain (i.e. erectile dysfunction, excessive menstrual bleeding); and one pseudo neurological symptom (i.e. blindness, seizures, paralysis). Patients with this disorder display a rather bland emotional response to these problems, do not seem particularly concerned with what these symptoms might mean, and seem to gain a good deal of attention and sympathy from their apparent discomfort. Most patients with this diagnosis are women from lower socioeconomic groups with little education. Somatization Disorder is very difficult to treat since the patient often has little insight or motivation to change. Case management is more often geared to reducing the inappropriate utilization of medical services.

Hypochondriasis

Hypochondriasis can be difficult to distinguish from Somatization Disorder for a naïve observer. Both disorders present to the examiner with physical concerns for which no actual physical basis can be found. Rather than focus their complaints primarily on a variety of symptoms, hypochondriacal patients misinterpret actual physical signs or symptoms they notice or experience as abnormal and the result of a disease or illness (Table 7.7). Despite any reassurance from medical personnel, patients persist in their belief and frequently experience significant

Table 7.7. Cardinal Signs and Symptoms: Hypochondriasis

- Belief that one has a disease based on misinterpretation of physical symptoms
- Belief is resistant to any reassurance
- Belief is not delusional, but causes impairment in daily functioning

Table 7.8. Cardinal Signs and Symptoms: Conversion Disorder

- Sensory or motor symptoms or deficits that suggest a neurological or general medical condition
- Psychological factors are judged to be associated with the deficits
- The deficits or symptoms are neither feigned or produced intentionally
- Symptoms cannot be fully explained by a general medical/substance use condition

depression and anxiety in relation to their intractable beliefs. A hypochondriacal individual may notice a mole on her hand and conclude that it is cancerous. These patients typically seek out a physician who, after appropriate evaluation, will reassure them that they are free of disease. Relieved initially, hypochondriacs will obsess over the possibility that the diagnosis was wrong and seek out other opinions. Emergency medical personnel may encounter individuals with this disorder who request assistance regularly, even chronically dialing 911. First Responders must keep in mind that even hypochondriacs may experience legitimate illness, and, consequently, they must always rule out medical causes before dismissing the complaints or referring the subjects to a mental health professional. Needless to say, hypochondriacs are very difficult to treat, and their disorders tend to be chronic in spite of medical or psychological intervention. In fact, the attention that a patient receives in seeking out medical treatment can be viewed as the reinforcement of a "sick role," a comfortable position for someone who needs to avoid the responsibility that a "healthy" person must shoulder.

Conversion Disorder

Similar to the Somatoform Disorders discussed above, *Conversion Disorder* also focuses on somatic symptoms and physical dysfunction without organic etiology to explain the problem (Table 7.8). However, the symptoms characteristically mimic neurological symptoms, including loss of sensory or motor functioning. Patients diagnosed with this disorder will develop symptoms such as blindness, deafness, fainting, seizures, or paralysis in some region of the body. The symptoms frequently emerge abruptly, often in response to some highly stressful or traumatic experience and may remit just as abruptly. Patients with the disorder often appear quite nonchalant about their impairment, in sharp contrast to the

---

BOX 7.5

Conversion Disorder

A police sergeant presented at a mental health center referred by an ophthalmologist complaining that he was unable to see anything but the largest objects. He was unable to drive, read or function on the job. His ophthalmologist reported that the patient had no physical evidence of any problem. Under hypnosis and with direct suggestion, he was able to read small print and function quite well, but when returned to normal consciousness, his problem returned. His reported history revealed that the officer had recently developed the problem and was particularly concerned because he was scheduled to take the qualification test to become a detective in the coming weeks. His problem had derailed that plan. Further exploration revealed that the officer was experiencing a great deal of marital conflict over financial problems and his wife had insisted that he advance himself in his department and become more financially secure. He related that he feared divorce if he did not accede to her wishes. The situation was complicated by the fact that he loved his job and did not want another position. It became clear after several sessions that the unconscious resolution to his conflict was the development of blindness and the socially acceptable excuse that he was unable to take the examination.

---

alarming reaction we might expect from an individual suddenly developing blindness or the inability to speak. This blasé attitude has been labeled "la belle indifference" and may serve as a helpful sign in distinguishing between conversion disorder and real neurological impairment which causes patients to express genuine concern over their symptoms. Another important distinction involves differentiating conversion disorder from malingering. Malingerers feign symptoms like blindness or paralysis for some immediate gain like monetary compensation or avoiding legal difficulties. They are always aware of their true motivations.

Individuals suffering from Conversion Disorder have typically experienced some overwhelming traumatic stress like witnessing a murder, narrowly escaping a fire, or being confronted with divorce papers from which actual escape is impossible or socially unacceptable. We speculate that the individual *unconsciously* converts their psychological conflicts and fears into physical symptoms. These symptoms enable them to at least temporarily avoid dealing with their conflicts and thereby help them avoid debilitating anxiety and emotional discomfort, all the time believing that they are physically ill. The symptoms will typically continue until the underlying problems can be addressed and resolved and the individual faces and deals with the emotional trauma. See Box 7.5 for a case study of Conversion Disorder.

Two other Somatoform Disorders are *Pain Disorder* and *Body Dysmorphic Disorder*. The latter involves the experience of pain in the absence of any organic basis or pain that is far in excess of what would be expected based on the patient's actual physical findings. Interestingly, pain clinics that treat these individuals have discovered that the majority of their patients, usually women, have a history of physical or sexual abuse. Psychologist Mary Koss' research found that these victims make twice as many visits to medical doctors as non-abused patients.

Body Dysmorphic Disorder involves a person's preoccupation with some imagined defect in appearance when, in fact, the person looks quite normal to any observer. Such patients constantly ruminate over the "imperfection" and experience significant distress as they check themselves in the mirror or avoid social contact, believing that everyone will be looking at them. Many go to extreme lengths to change their appearance and often undergo repeated plastic surgeries to correct the "problem."

DISSOCIATIVE DISORDERS

Everyone has had the experience of daydreaming in which they lose their awareness of their immediate surroundings and become caught up in a thought or some external distraction. During this experience they may lose track of time or even fail to hear someone calling to them. When this happens while driving and a person suddenly realizes that miles have passed without any conscious awareness, it can be quite disconcerting. Additionally, most individuals have had the experience of hearing very upsetting news about a death or serious illness and immediately feeling numb, confused, and disconnected from what was going on around them. Children who are repeatedly abused often learn to separate their mind from their body and dissociate so that they do not feel the pain. In all these cases, the individuals have experienced a mild form of *dissociation* that may involve an alteration in their memory, their perception of reality, and their sense of their own identity. In the most extreme cases that rise to the level of a disorder, these alterations are profound and significantly impair the persons' ability to function.

Dissociative Amnesia

Dissociative Amnesia involves the inability to remember important personal information that is usually related to some stressful or traumatic situation and cannot be explained by simple forgetting (Table 7.9). Dissociative amnesia must be differentiated from amnestic disorder that is always the result of a medical condition or the use of substances. In the case of dissociative amnesia, the individual psychologically "needs" to forget the trauma in order to avoid the emotional pain and disruption that would presumably arise from remembering it. Like conversion symptoms, the amnesia is not intentionally produced.

Table 7.9. Cardinal Signs and Symptoms: Dissociative Amnesia

* Episodes of inability to recall typically traumatic or stressful information that is beyond normal forgetting
* Not due to a general medical/substance use condition

Dissociative Fugue

Dissociative Fugue is a rather intriguing disorder that also involves loss of memory for one's past, but is primarily characterized by sudden travel away from one's home or work (Table 7.10). Individuals with this disorder may take on another identity and be unable to remember where they came from or why they are in a new location. The disorder often begins abruptly in response to some significant stress and ends abruptly as well. Some believe that sleepwalking is a Dissociate Fugue state.

Dissociative Identity Disorder

Dissociative Identity Disorder has been the topic of many books and movies over the years and represents one of the most controversial diagnoses in psychiatric literature (Table 7.11). It incorporates elements of both dissociative amnesia and fugue, but adds a dimension that involves the fragmentation of the patient's personality into two or more identities or *alters*. Originally labeled Multiple Personality Disorder, the diagnosis was changed to clarify that patients do not have several people inside of them. Rather, their identity has been dissociated or split off into fragments, each representing aspects of the person's traumatic history and conflicts. Alters may switch as one emerges to take control of the patient's behavior at some point, while remaining unknown to the other alters as well as to the host personality. These "amnestic barriers" protect the patient from awareness of their conflicts and past trauma. Many patients will have an alter that is very sexual and often presents as a prostitute. Another common alter serves as a protector. Many studies have found alters differing in voice tone, handwriting, and even physical characteristics like blood pressure and handedness.

Table 7.10. Cardinal Signs and Symptoms: Dissociative Fugue

- Sudden travel away from home or work with inability to remember one's past
- Confusion about personal identity or taking on a new identity
- Not due to a general medical/substance use condition

Table 7.11. Cardinal Signs and Symptoms: Dissociative Identity Disorder

- Presence of two or more identities or personality states
- At least two states recurrently take control of person's behavior
- Inability to remember important personal information that is beyond simple forgetting
- Not due to a general medical/substance use condition

Dissociative Identity Disorder is diagnosed primarily in women and is co-morbid with several other psychiatric disorders including Post Traumatic Stress Disorder, Complex PTSD, Borderline Personality Disorder, substance abuse, and depression, many of which share very similar symptoms. The disorder almost invariably is related to persistent and typically sadistic and inescapable sexual and physical abuse during childhood. Faced with intolerable abuse and no ability to escape, children may revert to fantasy and learn to "dissociate" from their immediate experience to relieve their psychological pain. This strategy seems to set the stage for the development of this fragmented identity that continues to protect patients from their past.

Treatment of DID is an incredibly complex endeavor. The most ambitious goal has been to reintegrate the personality and break down the amnestic barriers that prevent the patients from becoming aware of their trauma. More typically, clinicians help patients face the traumatic history, desensitize them to its effects and help them identify triggers that re-ignite their painful memories.

SUGGESTED READINGS

Andrews, G., Cramer, M., Crino, R., Hunt, C., Lampe, L. & Page, A. (2003). *The treatment of anxiety disorders*. New York: Cambridge University Press.

Barlow, D. H. (2002). *Anxiety and its disorders: The nature and treatment of anxiety and panic*. (2nd edn). New York: Guilford.

Barlow, D. H. & Durand, V. M. (2005). *Abnormal psychology: An integrative approach*. New York: Thomson Wadsworth.

Beck, A. T. & Emery, G. (1985). *Anxiety disorders and phobias: A cognitive perspective*. New York: Basic Books.

Breslau, N., Kessler, R. C., Chilcoat, H. D., Schultz, L. R., Davis, G. C., & Andreski, P. (1998). Trauma and posttraumatic stress disorder in the community: The 1996 Detroit Area Survey of Trauma. *Archives of general psychiatry, 55*, 626–632.

Cohen, L., Berzoff, J., & Elin, M. (Eds.). (1995). *Dissociative identity disorder. Theoretical and treatment controversies*. Northvale, NJ: Jason Aronson.

Craske, M. G. & Barlow, D. H. (2000). *Mastery of your anxiety and panic*. (3rd edn). New York: The Psychological Corporation.

Davidson, J. R. T. & Foa, E. B. (Eds.). (1993). *Posttraumatic stress disorder: DSM-IV and beyond*. Washington, DC: American Psychiatric Press.

Fritz, G. K., Fritsch, S., & Hagino, O. (1997). Somatoform disorders in children and adolescents: A review of the past 10 years. *Journal of the American Academy of Child and Adolescent Psychiatry, 36*, 1329 (10).

Grossman, D. (1995). *On killing: The psychological cost of learning to kill in war and society*. Boston, MA: Little, Brown and Company.

Haddock, D. B. (2001). *Dissociative identity disorder*. New York: McGraw-Hill Professional.

Heimberg, R. G., Liebowitz, M. R., Hope, D.A., & Schneier, F. R. (Eds.). (1995). *Social Phobia: Diagnosis, assessment and treatment*. New York: Guilford Press.

Hyman, B. M. & Pedrich, C. (2006). *Anxiety disorders*. Minneapolis: Twenty-First Century Books.

Kellner, R. (1986). *Somatization and hypochondriasis*. New York: Praeger.

Kluft, R. P. (1991). Multiple personality disorder. In A. Tasman and S. M. Goldfinger (Eds.). *American psychiatric press review of psychiatry*, Vol. 10. Washington, DC: American Psychiatric Press.

Krahauer, S. Y. (2001). *Treating dissociative identity disorder*. Routledge.

Lynn, S. J. & Rhue, J. W. (1994). *Dissociation: Clinical and theoretical perspectives*. New York: Guilford.

Mayou, R., Bass, C. N., & Sharpe, M. (Eds.). (1995). *Treatment of functional somatic symptoms*. Oxford: Oxford University Press.

McCann, I. L. & Pearlman, L. A. (1990). *Psychological trauma and the adult survivor: Theory, therapy and transformation*. New York: Bruner/Mazel.

Rapee, R. M. & Barlow, D. H. (Eds.). (1991). *Chronic anxiety: Generalized anxiety disorder, and mixed anxiety and depression*. New York: Guilford Press.

Ross, C. A. (1997). *Dissociative identity disorder: Diagnosis, clinical features, and the treatment of multiple personality*. (2nd edn). New York: John Wiley.

Saks, E. R. & Behnke, S. H. (1997). *Jekyll on trial: Multiple personality disorder and criminal law*. New York: New York University Press.

Steketee, G. S. (1996). *Treatment of obsessive-compulsive disorder*. New York: Guilford.

Stien, D. J. (Ed.). (2004). *Clinical manual of anxiety disorders*. Washington D.C: American Psychiatric Press.

Swinson, R. P., Antony, M. M., Rachman, S. & Richter, M. A. (Eds.). (1998). *Obsessive-compulsive disorder: Theory, research, and treatment*. New York: Guilford Press.

Thigpen, C. H. & Cleckley, H. M. (1957). *The three faces of Eve*. New York: McGraw-Hill.

Trimble, M. (2004). *Somatoform disorders*. New York: Cambridge University Press.

Van der Kolk, B. A. (Eds.). (1987). *Psychological trauma*. Washington, DC: American Psychiatric Press.

Van der Kolk, B. A., McFarlane, A. C., & Weisath, L. (1996). *Traumatic stress: The effects of overwhelming stress on mind, body and society*. New York: Guilford Press.

Walker, J. R., Norton, G. R., & Ross, C. A. (Eds.). (1991). *Panic disorder and agoraphobia: A comprehensive guide for the practitioner*. Pacific Grove, CA: Brooks/Cole.

Weintraub, M. I. (1983). *Hysterical conversion reactions: A clinical guide to diagnosis and treatment*. New York: SP Medical and Scientific Books.

CHAPTER 8

The Personality Disorders

All previous chapters exploring pathological mental disorders have represented symptom oriented conditions, often characterized by their intermittent course with periods of remission and exacerbation and described by clinicians as "medical conditions." Schizophrenia and bipolar illness, for instance, often develop in early adulthood, and result in acute periods of severe symptoms at different points in the course of the disorders that respond to therapeutic intervention, whether through medication or psychotherapy. The *DSM-IV-TR* lists these disorders on Axis I in the multiaxial system and notes that they are the focus of our clinical treatment. In contrast to the Axis I disorders described in earlier chapters, personality disorders are diagnosed on Axis II; they are always chronic, unremitting, develop in childhood and adolescence and are highly resistant to any kind of therapeutic intervention. Many clinical disorders, from major depression and panic disorder to substance use disorders, often affect more well- circumscribed areas of daily functioning than personality disorders that tend to impact every area of one's life. As one might expect, clinical disorders like depression, schizophrenia, or hypochondriasis cause the patient significant distress and psychological pain. In contrast, individuals diagnosed with a personality disorder are generally free of significant anxiety, depression, or other subjective distress, but more commonly cause conflict and distress to others who must interact with them. This is not to suggest that a person with a personality disorder never suffers from psychological pain. It is common that patients with such a diagnosis may also suffer from a clinical disorder like depression or alcoholism. Having both an Axis I and Axis II disorder generally will complicate the treatment process and result in a poorer prognosis. As we explore the nature and types of personality disorders, the difficulty of treating a patient with a co-morbid personality disorder will become more evident.

FROM PERSONALITY TRAIT TO PERSONALITY DISORDER

We are all familiar with the notion of *"personality"* as a constellation of psychological characteristics or traits that involve our behavioral predispositions to act in predictable ways across time and situations, and in multiple interpersonal roles. We commonly describe others as "kind," "perfectionistic," "manipulative," "hostile," "dependent," "quiet," "suspicious," or with a myriad of other adjectives that portray how the person typically thinks or acts in most situations. Any one of these traits might accurately describe a person at some point in time or in a specific situation, but only when they manifest themselves consistently can we conclude that they define a component of one's "personality." Unlike clinical symptoms, personality traits that comprise personality are always longstanding, extremely refractory to change, and are often difficult to measure objectively. Even more difficult is distinguishing between "normal" personality and a personality disorder.

Many experts agree that, even though DSM-IV-TR describes personality disorders as "all or nothing," that is, the individual either meets the criteria for the diagnosis or not, personality disorders may be viewed as extreme variations of normal personalities. At any point a person may view a co-worker as a bit overbearing, hostile, impulsive or dependent, looking to others to make decisions in stressful situations. These traits, however, may be situation specific and transient since the observer sees that this person is very composed, thoughtful and independent in most other circumstances. However, when the constellation of traits is inflexible regardless of the demands of the situation, occurs consistently and inflexibly over time and is maladaptive and self defeating, causing pain and discomfort to themselves and others, clinicians are likely to see the personality as "abnormal" and diagnose it as a personality disorder. The DSM-IV-TR lists ten personality disorders, several of which will have particular importance to First Responders who undoubtedly will encounter individuals with these disorders in the field.

Prevalence and Etiology

Because of the rather subjective nature of the personality disorder diagnosis and the fact that those diagnosed with one of the disorders do not typically present themselves to researchers or clinicians for evaluation or treatment, establishing accurate prevalence rates has been difficult. However, several researchers have published rates for each of the ten disorders, and the DSM-IV-TR has summarized the rates for all personality disorders at up to 2.5% of the general population, 10–30% of patients in inpatient settings, and 2% to 10% of patients in outpatient settings. However, according to the results of the 2001–2002 National Epidemiologic Survey on Alcohol and Related Conditions (NESARC) reported in the *Journal of Clinical Psychiatry* in 2004, an estimated 30.8 million American adults (14.8%) meet standard diagnostic criteria for at least one personality disorder as defined in the *DSM-IV-TR*.

The development of personality disorders involves a highly complex interplay between individuals' biology and their psychological, physical, and social environments. It is clearly not a linear process, but one that involves multiple, interactive determinants that influence and shape individuals from the beginning to the end of their lives. As they do with many other psychopathological disorders, experts agree that biology plays an important role in the development of personality disorders. Heredity is likely to represent a predisposition or diathesis to specific personality characteristics that will express themselves in response to certain environmental stressors and learning histories. Neurological "wiring" and the basic functional integrity of the central nervous system surely have an impact on how people interact with their world. "Temperament" represents the totality of biological contributions that the infant brings into the world that are manifested in patterns of unlearned behavioral dispositions like activity level, sleeping and eating patterns, and response to touch and holding. The development of personality disorders may involve not only the direct effects of children's temperaments, but what kind of response these dispositions elicit from significant others in their environment. Fussy, irritable infants might cause insecure mothers to reject these children and avoid holding or soothing them, while other caregivers may react in a supportive and reassuring way to the same children. These different interactions may contribute to early development of very different personality traits and, under the more negative parenting, ultimately to a personality disorder.

While biology plays a crucial role in the development of personality disorders, it is the impact of the psychological and physical environment with which it interacts that holds great interest for the professional as well as lay person. The quality of emotional support in the environment that protects the developing child from stress and anxiety, the opportunity to learn from others effective coping skills to deal with life, and the absence of traumatic experiences like physical and sexual abuse, early losses of caretakers, and serious medical illness will help to determine whether or not an individual develops a personality disorder. Being born to parents who themselves are not emotionally healthy, who use punitive or inconsistent discipline, and who create chronic family chaos is likely to result in the creation of impossible conditions to which a child must adapt. The consequence of this overwhelming stress may be the development of maladaptive behaviors and personality traits that may reduce the child's anxiety, but will continue to be used inappropriately to manage stress throughout the individual's life. The persistent and rigid personality style (i.e. personality disorder) that emerges elicits anger and other negative responses from others, thus reinforcing the self defeating pattern of behavior. What was adaptive in a child's early pathological environment, continues throughout adulthood when, in fact, it is no longer effective. It is the rigidity, persistence, and stability of such a pattern in the face of negative interpersonal consequences that define a personality disorder.

Explaining the pathological development of personality remains a highly speculative and theoretical enterprise since few empirical data exist to substantiate the actual etiology of personality disorders. Mental health professionals recognize, and lay persons intuitively know, that many individuals with devastating childhoods grow up to be healthy adults, while those blessed with apparently emotionally healthy environments develop serious personality pathology. The complexity of this process remains to be unraveled.

The *DSM-IV-TR* lists ten personality disorders that are grouped into three clusters, each of which shares some similar characteristics with others. The three groups can be described as the "Odd," the "Dramatic," and the "Anxious" clusters. The Odd cluster is composed of the Schizoid, Schizotypal, and Paranoid personality disorders; the Anxious cluster is composed of the Dependent, Obsessive Compulsive, and Avoidant personality disorders; and the Dramatic cluster contains the Histrionic, Narcissistic, Borderline and Anti-Social personality disorders. Each of these disorders will be described below.

THE ODD CLUSTER

Schizoid Personality Disorder

Law enforcement personnel will be familiar with the homeless individual who wanders the streets alone, never speaking to anyone neither involved with nor interested in any close relationships. It is likely that many of the homeless could be diagnosed as schizoid personalities who experience no pleasure in interpersonal relationships, avoid closeness with anyone, and engage exclusively in solitary activities. If officers were to engage such a person in conversation, they would find a very cold, detached and indifferent individual who would display little emotion and would be unlikely to respond to any praise or criticism that might be offered. Individuals with *Schizoid Personality* are not interested in sexual relationships and, in fact, experience little pleasure in any activity. When they are employed, it is likely to be in jobs with little interpersonal contact (Table 8.1).

The cause and development of all personality disorders remain complex and poorly understood areas. Theoretically, biological and psychosocial factors play a part in the development of schizoid pathology. Genetic loading or brain abnormalities may result in certain response tendencies that help to account for the individual's lack of emotional reactivity and social introversion. Schizoid personality disorder may be conceived as lying on a continuum from normal shyness and introversion

Table 8.1. Cardinal Signs and Symptoms: Schizoid Personality Disorder

- Does not enjoy close relationships
- Chooses solitary activities
- Little sexual interest in others
- Does not enjoy any activities
- Lacks close friends
- Indifferent to praise or criticism
- Cold, detached

to full blown schizophrenia, and differ genetically from schizophrenia in terms of the smaller number of genes the schizoid individual carries. Psychologically, one may speculate that infants with this temperament would be unresponsive to caretakers, would fail to form emotional attachments, and would reject loving parents through their apparent disinterest. Caretakers, in turn, failing to be reinforced for their attention, may begin to move away from these children, further isolating them and ultimately reinforcing their developing socially indifferent personality style. Pediatric psychiatrist Stella Chess demonstrated these behaviors in her longitudinal study of infant-caretaker relationships.

Treatment for schizoid personality usually focuses on the development of social skills and on exposing the patient to more interpersonal and social experiences. The basic problem, however, is the patient's lack of interest in and motivation for seeking treatment in the first place. As mentioned earlier, individuals with schizoid personality disorder are not totally immune from stressors in their lives and the development of Axis I disorders like psychotic or mood disorders. Under these circumstances, they are more likely to seek help and be willing to address their personality pathology.

Schizotypal Personality Disorder

Schizotypal Personality Disorder combines the major characteristic of the schizoid, namely the impaired capacity for and interest in emotional attachment to others, with unusual thinking and strange behavior. Along what is referred to as the "schizophrenic spectrum" or continuum of disorders, schizotypal personality lies closer to full blown schizophrenia than schizoid personality. Schizotypal personalities manifest a variety of "psychotic-like" thoughts and behaviors that border on schizophrenia, but typically are able to function without fully decompensating into the full schizophrenic syndrome. Individuals with this diagnosis often believe that others are "referring" to them in some way or making them the center of everyone's attention. Two individuals innocently talking, a child's laugh, or cars passing by on a street can be seen by schizotypal persons as having some special relevance to them. These *ideas of reference* are not necessarily fixed and intractable like delusions, and individuals may be able to acknowledge that their beliefs are not valid. Individuals with this disorder will engage in strange and magical thinking, abstract philosophical preoccupations and superstitious behavior. Persons may believe that they can read minds or influence the behavior of others through telepathy, mind reading, or witchcraft. Perceptual distortions are common in which patients may experience "illusions" or misperceptions related to the environment or to their own bodies. Depersonalized feelings or déjà vu experiences border on, but are not as severe as, the clearly false sensations called hallucinations that reflect the psychotic process in schizophrenia.

When interviewing individuals with schizotypal personality, a First Responder will notice that their speech is quite difficult to follow, rambling and circumstantial with irrelevant details and abstract references that are vague and metaphorical. They may be quite suspicious of interviewers' motives and hold paranoid ideas that First Responders are part of a subtle conspiracy trying to entrap them. Consequently, they will often display a significant degree of social anxiety for fear of what might happen should they become too close or too familiar. Their behavior and appearance are often strange and inappropriate, with clothing poorly coordinated and makeup excessive (Table 8.2).

To understand the development and etiology of the Schizotypal Personality Disorder, one must return to the notion of the schizophrenic spectrum of disorders. Researchers have increasing empirical support that this disorder arises from the basic genetic underpinnings, referred to as the *schizotype*, which gives rise to schizophrenia. The extent and type of the genetic loading, in combination with a variety of psychological and environmental factors, will determine which of the spectrum disorders will be expressed. Early life experiences including parental indifference and rejection, disordered and confusing communication from caretakers, physical and sexual abuse, as well as physical illness, may play a role in the development of the personality disorder as it does in schizophrenia.

Table 8.2. Cardinal Signs and Symptoms: Schizotypal Personality Disorder

- Ideas of reference
- Odd, superstitious or magical beliefs
- Strange perceptual experiences
- Odd thinking and speech
- Paranoid
- Inappropriate affect
- Odd behavior or appearance
- Few friends
- Heightened social anxiety

Not surprisingly, treatment for Schizotypal Personality is exceedingly problematic. The individual's fundamental impairment in interpersonal relating, suspiciousness, and social anxiety result in significant difficulty in establishing a therapeutic relationship. The focus of treatment ideally surrounds increasing trust and value in the interpersonal/social world through a positive relationship with the therapist. Social skills training and medication management to treat the positive psychotic-like symptoms, as well as depression and anxiety, are typically employed.

Paranoid Personality Disorder

Frequently police officers have been called to the home of angry residents who claim their neighbors have been harassing them or in some way violating their rights. Callers might complain that their neighbor intentionally placed their garbage cans on the their property, played music too loudly in order to maliciously keep the complainant awake at night, or insist that their pet was ill because the neighbors poisoned the innocent animal. An officer called to a home where domestic violence has occurred may encounter an irate husband who insists that his wife has been cheating on him. Upon questioning the husband, the officer hears that he insists that his evidence is the expression on his wife's face whenever she meets with his son's school teacher. He offers no other evidence. In both these cases, the individual in question might suffer from *Paranoid Personality Disorder*.

This personality type is characterized by pervasive distrust and suspicion of others. Paranoid personalities display a profound lack of trust in everyone, believing everyone's motives are hostile and designed to take advantage of them. No one can be trusted; even loyalty of their closest friends or relatives cannot be taken for granted, since paranoids fear exposure of any personal vulnerability will be exploited and used against them. In order to guard against attack from others, paranoid individuals will be constantly vigilant, searching the environment for any indication that threats are imminent. In their investigation, officers in the cases described above would find very guarded, hostile, rigid and self righteous individuals who would challenge any attempt to evaluate the reality of their allegations. Rather, they would look for the minutest details in the situation that would confirm their paranoid suspicions. Paranoid personalities "see what they believe" rather than "believe what they see."

Some individuals diagnosed as paranoid personalities may present as quite grandiose and arrogant as a way to protect their very fragile self-esteem. Others may try to control their threatening world by going on the offense, challenging societal rules and often becoming quite litigious, suing anyone who they feel has wronged them (Table 8.3).

The development of the Paranoid Personality remains, like many of the personality disorders, complex and without much empirical

Table 8.3. Cardinal Signs and Symptoms: Paranoid Personality Disorder

- Suspicious without cause of others harming or deceiving them
- Concerned over loyalty and trustworthiness of associates and friends
- Cannot confide in others for fear of being harmed
- Reads hidden threatening meaning into harmless situations
- Bears grudges
- Sees attacks on themselves that others
- Suspicious of fidelity of partner or spouse

support. Biological and genetic antecedents have not been clearly established, although the more severe forms of the disorder may have some relationship to schizophrenia and delusional disorder like the schizoid and schizotypal types, the paranoid may experience much hostility, rejection, and unreasonable punishment as a child. Unpredictable environments characterized by unavailable caretakers who use inconsistent and sometimes sadistic discipline may set the stage for the child's inability to develop trust in what is perceived as a hostile world.

As one might expect, paranoid personalities are unlikely to seek treatment of their personality style. If they are seen at all, they will be referred by the police, employers, or spouses who have been affected by their behavior. The initial response of such a patient will be to project the blame for the problem on the other person, alleging, for instance, a conspiracy of police, unfair labor practices, or marital infidelity. Support and a non-evaluative and non-confrontational therapeutic style are critical if any relationship can be established. Cognitive therapy aimed at helping patients to objectively evaluate their concerns, developing problem-solving skills for specific situations, and even relaxation training to help deal with their fears and anxiety can be helpful. Ideally, the ultimate goal is to assist paranoid persons in addressing their own internal insecurities and fears that have led to their defensive and self defeating personality style.

THE ANXIOUS CLUSTER

Avoidant Personality Disorder

It is unlikely that a person with an *Avoidant Personality Disorder* would come to the attention of law enforcement personnel. These individuals are characterized as deeply insecure, socially inhibited and fearful of any negative evaluation. The thought of acting out, behaving in an aggressive or competitive manner, or challenging authority would cause them great anxiety, shame, and humiliation. Individuals with this personality disorder rarely venture out into the social world for fear of criticism and rejection. Believing that they are fundamentally inferior, inept, and inadequate, they avoid any situation in which

Table 8.4. Cardinal Signs and Symptoms: Avoidant Personality Disorder

- Avoids employment that requires much interpersonal contact for fear of criticism or disapproval
- Will not be involved with others unless certain of acceptance
- Restrained with intimate relationships fearing ridicule
- Fears being criticized in social situations
- Inhibited interpersonally based on feeling inadequate
- Believes they are socially inadequate and inferior
- Avoids risk-taking fearing embarrassment

they might face rejection or judgment and expose themselves only when they feel absolutely reassured and safe. As a result, they are likely to have few friends who can meet this test. Unlike the Schizoid Personality who has no interest in social or emotional involvement with others, the avoidant individual may crave closeness and attention from others, but withdraw from such risks, inhibit their desire for intimacy, and retreat to their private safe harbor.

Individuals diagnosed with Avoidant Personality Disorder may often find themselves in work that is far below their potential. In order to avoid evaluation of their performance, they tend to seek work environments with few demands and little interpersonal contact. Their goal is to bring as little attention to themselves as possible (Table 8.4).

To understand the origins and development of the Avoidant Personality we again look to its psychobiological and environmental roots. A biologically based temperament with a low threshold for stress and anxiety may result in a child who is fearful, insecure, and reticent to become close with others or experiment with new situations. When caretakers react to this behavioral style, they may feel frustrated with their children's failure to respond to new challenges and communicate this disappointment to the children. Gradually, this negative feedback becomes internalized as a sign of rejection, resulting in feelings of shame and inadequacy. Chaotic and disruptive influences during children's development including physical or sexual abuse or even the unexpected death of a parent may further reinforce a belief that they are worthless and defective. This reciprocal interaction between biological and psychological influences remains speculative without much empirical support.

Treatment of Avoidant Personality Disorder is difficult and requires a highly supportive and non-evaluative therapeutic relationship. Like the treatment of social phobia with which it is frequently co-morbid, desensitizing patients to social situations by exposing them gradually to a variety of social environments has been helpful. Cognitive therapy aimed at challenging their beliefs about self worth and their catastrophic fears of rejection and criticism may help to reduce anxiety and feelings of embarrassment. Improving patients' social skills through role-playing has also been useful.

Dependent Personality Disorder

While it is normal and healthy to depend on others in our life to meet many of our emotional and practical needs, and equally appropriate and desirable to sacrifice at times for the benefit of those we care about, those who have *Dependent Personality Disorder* have a pathological tendency to do both. That is, dependent personalities look to others to be taken care of, feeling helpless and fearful of managing their lives independently. In order to secure the assistance from others for the smallest task or decision, dependent individuals will behave in a highly submissive, pleasing and deferent manner to insure that no one will reject them or refuse to offer nurturance and support. This style is in contrast to persons with avoidant personality who also feel inadequate and need constant reassurance, but manages their struggles by withdrawing from interpersonal relationships. Dependent individuals have no belief in their ability to manage their own lives, no willingness to make decisions without reassurance from others or to assume responsibility for many areas of their lives. They may refuse to learn the necessary skills that are required of an adult and basically arrange their lives in such a way that others are forced to make decisions for them. Choices surrounding work, school, financial matters, or living arrangements are left to others.

Dependent personalities live in fear of separation and abandonment. As a result of their implicit and often manipulative demands to be cared for by others and the resulting clingy nature of their interpersonal style, those on whom they are dependent often become intolerant and ultimately end the relationship. Dependent individuals are left feeling helpless, unable to care for themselves and desperate to find a replacement to rescue them from the perceived loss. In effect, it is as if dependent persons seek to return to or perhaps never leave the utter dependence and helplessness of their childhood (Table 8.5).

Researchers and clinicians speculate that individuals diagnosed with Dependent Personality Disorder have childhood histories characterized by overprotection and overindulgence by parents who may even discourage independence and autonomy as children develop. By addressing

Table 8.5. Cardinal Signs and Symptoms: Dependent Personality Disorder

- Requires excessive reassurance in order to make everyday decisions
- Looks to others to take responsibility for major areas of life
- Cannot disagree with others fearing loss of support
- Cannot initiate activities independently
- Goes to great lengths to insure support from others
- Uncomfortable being alone fearing that they will be unable to care for themselves
- Seeks immediately to replace any lost relationship
- Fears being left to care for themselves

every need the children have in spite of their ability to meet it independently, by communicating that children cannot face the world without their assistance, and by refusing to allow developing children to take risks, explore the environment on their own, or learn new competencies without fear of some "danger," parents set the stage for dependent pathology. The result leads to the failure of children to develop strong personal identities and to the development of the belief that they are helpless, unable to fend for themselves, and vulnerable to abandonment.

Unlike individuals with several other personality disorders, dependent personalities are likely to benefit from psychotherapy. The quality of the therapeutic relationship is critical, and the support and nurturance the patient receives are consistent with their needs for guidance and reassurance. At some point, however, therapists must help patients develop the insight and skills to handle their lives more independently. Cognitive therapy aimed at altering many of their irrational beliefs regarding their helplessness, as well as assertive training geared to improving interpersonal effectiveness and the ability for self representation, are effective tools in addressing dependent psychopathology.

Obsessive-Compulsive Personality Disorder

Many First Responders will recognize micromanaging sergeants who scrupulously check each accident report to insure that the geographical location of the accident being investigated is spelled correctly, that each blank on the report is filled in properly, and that the report covers the most insignificant details. When they discover some "imperfection," supervisors may become punitive and condescending to the officer, inflexible in dealing with the rules and regulations of the department that they believe must be followed. It is also likely that sergeants might be extremely dedicated to their jobs, to the exclusion of family and personal needs, and unwilling to trust subordinates with the responsibility of independently doing their jobs. Such a style is consistent with an *Obsessive-Compulsive Personality Disorder*.

Compulsives are focused on details, order, and organization in their daily lives, to the extent that in addressing any problem, they "cannot see the forest for the trees." They insist on perfection, from themselves as well as others, and become irritated and judgmental when others do not conform to their rules, regulations, and expectations. Fearing that others will not perform up to their unreasonably rigid standards, compulsive individuals will refuse to give others any responsibility or delegate tasks to subordinates. They fear to do so might result in condemnation and punishment from superiors. To avoid such a fate, compulsives are likely to be very deferential and supportive with their bosses from whom they seem to gain derivative power and authority, ultimately to be imposed on their subordinates. Unfortunately, faced with total responsibility to complete a task that must meet exacting standards, work often remains uncompleted or requires the individual to work to the point where there is no time for family, friends, and personal pleasures.

While, on the surface, compulsives appear to be "good, upstanding" individuals, their personality is characterized by very rigid, stubborn traits that make it difficult to work with or relate to them unless one is willing to submit to their uncompromising standards. This rigidity extends to their ethics and values and often characterizes moralistic, religious leaders. They are dogmatic in their beliefs, self righteous, and typically unwilling to be charitable when dealing with others' failings. Their tendency to punish themselves for any loss of control or imperfection is easily projected onto anyone who "misses a step." In everyday terms, the obsessive-compulsive person is a "control freak!" (Table 8.6).

The development of this disorder may have its roots in early childhood, particularly in the children's relationship with their parents. Rigid, cold and over controlling parents may demand perfection and adherence to rules that ignore the emotional needs and individuality of the child. Children may be exposed to expectations from parents for responsibility and deference that ignore and challenge their growing need for independence and autonomy. They are faced with a conflict between conforming to the demands of their parents in order to insure and obtain their love and approval and the need for independence and autonomy so critical in psychological development. This "no win" situation leaves developing children ambivalent, guilt-ridden and angry. As their personalities develop, they learn to find acceptance and approval from others in rigid adherence to rules and perfection, feel the need to be very responsible, yet display their anger and frustration through their over-control and critical demands displaced onto others. Compulsives are haunted by the "tyranny of the shoulds," a set of beliefs that reflect a world of all good and all bad with no room for emotion, doubt or weakness. When faced with the inevitable ambiguity of life, they experience anxiety and fear until they can establish a set of rules that point them to the "right" way in every decision.

Psychotherapy is a difficult endeavor for individuals with Obsessive-Compulsive Disorder. It represents for compulsive patients the task of

Table 8.6. Cardinal Signs and Symptoms: Obsessive Compulsive Personality Disorder

- Preoccupied with details and order
- Perfectionistic
- Excessively devoted to work to exclusion of leisure and friendships
- Over conscientious and rigid regarding morality and ethics
- Hoards worthless objects
- Unable to delegate tasks to others without micromanaging
- Miserly
- Rigid and stubborn

developing a relationship with an individual who is "in control" and who seeks to assist them in exploring emotions and beliefs with the goal of personality change. Experiencing emotions and abandoning old beliefs represent a true loss of control for compulsives who find comfort in rational, logical solutions to problems and in rigidly maintaining their own way of doing things. Nevertheless, they may find help in developing insight into how their perfectionism developed through an exploration of their developmental history and through the experience of relating to a therapist who makes no demands on them, offers no critical judgments of their behavior and unconditionally accepts them. Cognitive behavior therapy addressing their irrational beliefs and expectations as well as tension reduction procedures may also be helpful.

THE DRAMATIC CLUSTER

Histrionic Personality Disorder

While the obsessive-compulsive persons live their lives focused on details, rules, schedules, and rigid adherence to logic and moral absolutes, individuals with *Histrionic Personality Disorder* function in a world that they view in a highly emotional and impressionistic manner with little or no attention to "boring" facts and details or the careful analysis of the complexities of life. Emotions are superficial, constantly changing, and expressed in very dramatic ways. Histrionics' speech is typically vague, lacking in specifics and characterized by "glittering generalities" and exaggeration. Feelings seem to change like "shifting sands," and others begin to experience histrionics' emotional reactions as empty and inauthentic. This dramatic style is geared to drawing attention to themselves, striving constantly to be the focus of everyone's interest. Histrionic personalities, a type typically but not always diagnosed in women, will use their physical appearance, including their dress, makeup, and emotionality to interest others and gain their validation and approval. Histrionic individuals feel that they must be interesting and attractive to others and will use sexually seductive and alluring behavior to insure that attention. Interpersonal relationships are quite fleeting and unstable since histrionic people become bored very quickly. After the initial maneuvers to attract another's interest or curiosity has been achieved, histrionic persons have little interest or substance left to sustain a meaningful relationship. In spite of this, if they fail to gain the approval and praise that they crave from others, they are likely to become frustrated and angry (Table 8.7).

The early childhood of budding histrionics is often characterized by caretakers inconsistently acknowledging and validating only the "cute" behavior and engaging personal qualities they admire. Never being able to count on approval for the same behavior, these children begin to try harder and in more attention-seeking ways to insure the love they desire

Table 8.7. Cardinal Signs and Symptoms: Histrionic Personality Disorder

- Must be the center of attention
- Sexually seductive and provocative behavior with others
- Shifting and shallow expression of emotions
- Uses physical appearance to attract attention
- Vague and impressionistic speech
- Self dramatizing
- Highly suggestible
- Exaggerates degree of intimacy in relationships

from their parents. Sexual grooming behavior taught to young girls by pedophiles and incest fathers often continues into adolescence and adulthood. As young girls, in particular, reach adolescence and begin to recognize their own sexuality, socially approved attempts to secure love and attention, especially from males, reinforce this behavior and, consequently, the girls become more seductive and sexual for approval. As this strategy of attention-getting becomes increasingly more focused on superficial, often physical qualities, to the exclusion of more substantial values and competencies, these individuals internalize a self concept that leaves them feeling like a "pretty shell" that is empty inside. Many child beauty queens display these feelings. As women they develop the belief that the only way they can overcome their low self-esteem and feelings of inadequacy is through these exaggerated attention-seeking maneuvers that interest and intrigue others. Histrionic personalities protect themselves from awareness of their emptiness and sadness through their inattention to detail, refusal to look within themselves, and impressionistic style.

Psychotherapy for histrionic personality disorder is often focused on helping patients become more aware of their interpersonal behavior and their excessive need for attention. The therapist attempts to focus individuals on thinking rather than feeling, careful problem-solving rather than impulsive emotional reactions, and on exploring aspects of their personality that can enrich their identity beyond physical appearance and superficial charm. Feminist therapy helps women understand the social approval they obtain with seductive behavior and offers suggestions to alter these strategies in order to establish better relationships. Therapists seek to reinforce appropriate interactions during therapy and discourage histrionics' attempts to gain approval and support through seductive behavior with the therapist. The ultimate goals involve increasing self-esteem and confidence in their ability to be secure and loved without resorting to old attention-getting behavior.

Narcissistic Personality Disorder

In dealing with individuals with a narcissistic personality, one is immediately struck with their arrogance, inflated sense of their importance,

Table 8.8. Cardinal Signs and Symptoms: Narcissistic
Personality Disorder

- Grandiose sense of self importance
- Fantasizes about power and success
- Believes that they are "special"
- Demands admiration
- Sense of entitlement
- Exploits others
- Lacks empathy
- Envious of others
- Arrogant

---

and lack of empathy or sensitivity to the needs of others. Their grandiosity manifests itself in beliefs about unlimited success in all their endeavors and an expectation that others must treat them with special care and consideration, not holding them to the rules and regulations that ordinary people must abide by. The failure of others to appreciate their "specialness" can lead narcissists to angry outbursts, beliefs that only other special people could possibly understand their importance, or the assertion that others are simply envious of their achievement. It is not uncommon that, when faced with a severe blow to their self image, that is, a narcissistic injury, they can become quite depressed. Narcissistic individuals deal with other people as objects that are available to be exploited and used to meet their excessive needs for admiration. When faced with legitimate competition from another person, narcissistic individuals are likely to become quite envious in sharing the limelight (Table 8.8).

Theorists and clinicians offer several explanations regarding the development of narcissistic personality, some suggesting a failure of parents to offer opportunities to the child to learn empathy for others and a realistic appraisal of themselves. In some cases parents may so completely adore and worship their child that the child fails to appreciate that others in their world have separate feelings, desires, and beliefs, as well as importance in their own right. When parents continue to indulge their children's every wish, fail to set appropriate boundaries, or to teach their children that other people matter too, children grow up to become egocentric adults expecting others to admire and worship them as their parents did. Other theorists emphasize the defensive role of the narcissistic personality that serves to compensate for these individuals' underlying feelings of low self esteem and feelings of inadequacy.

Of particular interest to a First Responder who must function in a hierarchical organizational structure is a narcissistic chief or lieutenant who is expansive and grandiose and who demands unqualified obedience and admiration from his or her personnel. Individuals with such a personality type are impervious to feedback, tend to distort facts to fit their view of reality, and often will abuse their power.

In the unlikely event that persons with *Narcissistic Personality Disorder* seek psychological treatment, the presenting complaints typically center around feelings of disappointment and often rage that they have not been recognized as "special" or afforded the recognition they deserve. This interpersonal "injury" may lead them to feel depressed, empty, inadequate and searching for a therapist to re-install their sagging self-esteem. More typically, however, narcissists do not feel the need for treatment and generally function adequately, often at the expense of others whom they exploit.

Borderline Personality Disorder

Individuals diagnosed with *Borderline Personality Disorder* (BPD) display a complex array of behaviors and personality traits that combine elements of several Axis II disorders in the "dramatic" cluster, as well as symptoms associated with Axis I pathology, including depression, bipolar disorder, and post traumatic stress disorder. As a result, borderline pathology represents one of the most emotionally disruptive personality disorders and one that mental health professionals find most challenging to treat.

Probably one of the most obvious characteristics of the borderline is the marked instability and turmoil in their interpersonal relationships. These individuals will often seek intense emotional involvement with another person, becoming clingy, highly dependent and initially prone to idealizing them. The same individual who at one moment was idealized, loved and adored can quickly become devalued and hated when the borderline individual perceives some interpersonal slight or rejection. Unable to view themselves or others as an integrated mix of good and imperfect traits, the borderline thinks in dichotomous terms of all good and all bad, with nothing in between.

The instability in relationships is also manifested in borderline individuals' chronic fear of, and attempts to avoid, abandonment. As a result, they will have difficulty in maintaining appropriate boundaries with, and establishing realistic expectations of, others, making excessive demands for time, reassurance, and love. When these demands are not met, borderline individuals will often resort to impulsive behaviors including suicidal threats or gestures, substance abuse, and self-mutilation as a means to regulate their emotional turmoil, especially their anger and rage. Not infrequently this rage will also be directed to the once idealized persons who have "abandoned" them. Some will remember how this dynamic unfolds when the central character in the film "Fatal Attraction" played by Glenn Close is rejected and "abandoned" by her casual lover, played by Michael Douglas. Also central to borderline pathology is the disturbance of the individual's identity. While most of us have a clear and stable sense of our beliefs, values and attitudes, borderline individuals struggle with a constantly changing and porous self image. Changing jobs, immersing themselves impulsively and briefly in different hobbies, or frequently adopting different styles of dress reflect a very unstable sense of self.

Borderline patients will often complain of intense feelings of depression, emptiness, and irritability that are often transient, leaving them tossed about in emotional storms that come and go, often depending on the stress in their interpersonal relationships. Added to these emotional struggles are stress related paranoid thinking and dissociative experiences. Patients will complain that others are trying to hurt them and will describe "out of body" experiences or fears that they are not "real" or are no longer able to "feel." Sometimes they deal with this dissociative symptom by cutting themselves in order to feel something, even if it is pain. BPD is often confused with complex PTSD that shares many of the same personality traits, but arises from early and continued abuse. This is discussed in Chapter 10 (Table 8.9).

As with most of the personality disorders, theorists, researchers, and clinicians search for the etiology of the borderline character from both biological and psychological domains. While many theories have been developed, the actual development of borderline personality, like the other personality disorders, remains highly complex and speculative. The fact that emotional instability and mood disturbance are so central to the disorder has raised the possibility that biological factors may play a central role. Many theorists have suggested that borderline personality may be a form of depression or bipolar disorder and consequently have suggested the importance of an inherited trait or disposition that interacts with environmental and psychosocial factors to produce the personality style. Temperament characterized by impulsivity, hypersensitivity to stimulation, and irritability may interact with ineffective parenting to produce the characteristic personality pathology.

Perhaps the most detailed and complex theories of the etiology have been presented by psychodynamic authors who emphasize the inability of infants to develop a psychic structure and ego functions that enabled them to separate psychologically from their caretakers and develop a

Table 8.9. Cardinal Signs and Symptoms: Borderline Personality Disorder

- Frantic efforts to avoid abandonment
- Unstable, intense interpersonal relationships characterized by extremes of idealizing and devaluing others
- Identity disturbance
- Impulsivity that is self destructive including sex or substance abuse
- Suicidal gestures or self mutilation
- Affective instability that is transitory
- Feelings of emptiness
- Intense, inappropriate anger outbursts
- Transient paranoid or dissociative symptoms

separate and stable identity. From this dynamic perspective, the borderline personality lies somewhere between the "neurotic" and "psychotic"
levels of functioning. Most researchers underscore the role of an early
chaotic family environment characterized by family violence, substance
abuse, and anti-social behavior. Additionally, the frequency of sexual
and physical abuse of these individuals is high, along with parental neglect and abandonment. The predominance of sexual and physical
trauma in the borderline's history with that precipitating post traumatic
stress disorder has raised the possibility that these may be identical
disorders since they present with very similar symptom constellations.

Therapy for borderline patients is very difficult and typically long
term. The nature of their interpersonal difficulties, their inability
to develop clear interpersonal boundaries, and their tendency to see
relationships as either all good or all bad make therapy a treacherous
endeavor for the clinician. At one moment, the therapist may be perceived by the patient as a savior and, at the next, as an uncaring hurtful
person. Managing this "splitting" effectively, setting clear boundaries,
and maintaining an empathic, supportive, and caring balance with gen-
tle confrontation are all critical to successful therapy. A relatively new
treatment approach called Dialectical Behavior Therapy, developed by
Marcia Linehan, focuses on helping the patient to cope more effectively
with day to day stressors, and has proven quite successful with this
population. Of course, antidepressant medication, atypical anti-psychotic
drugs as well as mood stabilizers like lithium and Trileptal are employed
to address the often dramatic mood instability that accompanies not
only borderline personality but Major Depression and BiPolar Disorder,
diagnoses that are often co-morbid with borderline pathology.

Anti-Social Personality Disorder

Of all the personality disorders that have been presented, law enforcement personnel will have the most contact and experience with the anti-
social type. It is by far the most "dramatic" and combines characteristics
of the manipulative histrionic, the suspicious paranoid, the impulsive,
angry borderline, and the entitled narcissist. The anti-social personality
adds other key ingredients involving the absence of a conscience and a
history of violations of society's laws and mores. In his 1993 text entitled
*Without Conscience: The Disturbing World of the Psychopaths Among
Us*, Robert Hare eloquently describes psychopaths as "social predators
who charm, manipulate, and ruthlessly plow their way through life, leaving a broad trail of broken hearts, shattered expectations, and empty wal-
lets. Completely lacking in conscience and empathy, they selfishly take
what they want and do so as they please, violating social norms and
expectations without the slightest sense of guilt or regret."

First Responders will recognize anti-social individuals as those who
continuously break the law, lie and con others for their own needs, and
fail to see long-term consequences of their behavior, impulsively seeking

more immediate gratification. These individuals are typically angry and aggressive, irresponsible in work and interpersonal relationships, and deficient in experiencing guilt or remorse for their behavior. Many individuals well known in the criminal justice system come to mind who most dramatically meet these criteria: John Dillinger, John Wayne Gacy, Richard Speck, Ted Bundy, John Gotti, and Charles Manson. However, most of these "social predators" fly under the radar in our daily lives and may never come to the attention of law enforcement personnel.

One of the confusing issues surrounding this personality disorder is the variety of labels that have been employed to describe it. In addition to anti-social personality, "moral insanity," "sociopathy," and "psychopathy," as well as the more common law enforcement terms of "criminality" and "delinquency," have been used in the literature. While there is considerable overlap among these labels, there are significant differences among them both theoretically and empirically.

Three of the most commonly used terms in the psychiatric and criminal justice literature are *"psychopath," "anti-social personality disorder,"* and *"criminality."* The first label was most carefully defined by a psychiatrist named Hervey Cleckley who published a seminal work in 1941 on this psychopathy in a text entitled *The Mask of Sanity*. The anti-social personality disorder was initially described in the 1980 publication of the *DSM*. In its current edition, this volume lists very specific criteria to be used by the mental health establishment in diagnosing the disorder and anti-social personality is the term that enjoys the most currency today. Finally, "criminality" represents a common term used by law enforcement professionals and lay people alike. These three labels emphasize different aspects of this characterologically disturbed individual. Cleckley emphasized the underlying personality traits of the "psychopath," while the criteria of the *DSM-IV-TR* focus on the observable behaviors of the anti-social personality that can be readily identified by clinicians. "Criminal" simply defines an individual who breaks the law.

Cleckley described the "psychopath" as an individual who can appear quite "normal" to the casual observer and may never have come into contact with the criminal justice system. However, beneath this "normal" and often charming facade or "mask of sanity" lies an individual who has never developed a conscience and cannot experience remorse, shame, or empathy for others or experience adequate emotional responsiveness. These individuals do not experience anxiety, worry or depression. When law enforcement personnel encounter psychopaths who appear to be anxious, fearful, or sad, it is in most instances the result of being caught. When they can blame others for their misdeeds, avoid punishment, or in some manner escape consequences for their behavior, any emotional distress they may have experienced dissipates quickly. These individuals fail to learn from experience, have poor judgment, are unable to love, and are typically pathological liars. Basing his work on Cleckley's original criteria, Robert Hare developed a psychopathy checklist that is presented in Box 8.1

BOX 8.1

Robert Hare's 1991 Checklist based on Cleckley's (1941) Criteria for Psychopathy

- Glib and superficial charm
- Grandiose self worth
- Need for stimulation or proneness to boredom
- Pathological lying
- Conning and manipulativeness
- Lack of remorse or guilt
- Shallow affect
- Callousness and lack of empathy
- Parasitic lifestyle
- Poor behavioral controls
- Promiscuous sexual behavior
- Early behavior problems
- Lack of realistic, long term, goals
- Impulsivity
- Irresponsibility
- Failure to accept responsibility for own actions
- Many short-term marital relationships
- Juvenile delinquency
- Revocation of conditional release
- Criminal versatility

Table 8.10. Cardinal Signs and Symptoms: Anti-Social Personality Disorder

- Engages in unlawful behavior
- Deceitfulness
- Impulsivity
- Aggressiveness
- Disregard for safety of others
- Irresponsibility
- Lack of remorse

The individual diagnosed with Anti-Social Personality Disorder may often meet many of Cleckley's criteria for psychopathy, but additionally has engaged in unlawful, aggressive or irritable behavior. Key signs and symptoms of the DSM-IV-TR Anti-Social Personality Disorder are presented in Table 8.10.

Criminality defines the tendency to break the law without necessarily inferring any other underlying personality or behavioral characteristics. Some theorists have suggested that, if these individuals have no motivation to exert interpersonal control over another person, but are only interested in personal gain, they would not be diagnosed anti-social personality. Obviously, there is very significant overlap among these three constructs, but notwithstanding some of the valid theoretical differences that have been established in the literature, the choice of terms to describe this type of individual is often arbitrary and based on the preference of the diagnostician. For the purposes of this chapter, we will use the current *DSM-IV-TR* label of Anti-Social Personality.

Research addressing the development and etiology of the anti-social personality has been interesting and often focused on biological, genetic, and psychological variables. In research designed similarly to that involving schizophrenia and mood disorders, family, adoption and twin studies point to a very strong influence of genetics on the development of anti-social and criminal behavior. Some theories addressing neurobiological influences suggest that anti-social personalities have low levels of cortical arousal that they cope with by seeking out highly sensational and risky situations that excite them and counter their feelings of boredom. However, as with schizophrenia or mood disorders, genetics and biology cannot account for all the influences. While these individuals may inherit strong temperamental qualities including aggressiveness, lack of fear, impulsivity, and high sensation seeking, how the environment and, in particular, their parents deal with these response styles will be critical in determining their fate. Effective limit setting, sound, consistent discipline and loving, sensitive parents may mold that temperament in positive ways, while neglectful, controlling, punitive or abusive parents may insure that the genetic predisposition will be manifested in criminal behavior. Given these circumstances, developing children may never learn to manage their aggressive tendencies. On the contrary, the social models that they have encountered may have taught them the value of hostile behavior in accomplishing their goals and reinforced the need to be independent from any social or authoritarian control. Their attention becomes fixed on achieving immediate gratification at all costs.

Psychotherapeutic treatment of the anti-social personality is unlikely to be successful. In the absence of any emotional discomfort that so often motivates change in most individuals, persons with this diagnosis see no reason to change their behavior. Typically referred by significant others in their lives or the justice system, these patients will con and manipulate the clinician in order to gain the control in the relationship. They can be superficially cooperative, deferent and ingratiating in their interactions or openly intimidating to the interviewer, but never open, remorseful or insightful about their behavior. Clinicians and researchers in this area are more likely to focus on prevention programs addressing adolescent conduct disorders that serve as the precursors to a full blown disorder. Focusing on enhancing teenagers' social skills, and their abilities to manage conflict, and addressing problems of early alcohol and drug abuse, may prove to make an impact on their future behavior. In addition, research into parent training and interventions to enhance family functioning in early childhood may also have some long-range benefits.

SUGGESTED READINGS

Baltes, M. M. (1996). *The many faces of dependency in old age*. New York: Cambridge University Press.

Beck, A. T., Freeman, A. F., & Davis, D. (2003). *Cognitive therapy of personality disorders*. (2nd edn). New York: Guilford Press.

Benjamin, L. S. (1993). *Interpersonal diagnosis and treatment of personality disorders*. New York: Guilford Press.

Bleiberg, E. (2004) *Treating personality disorders in children and adolescents: A relational approach*. New York: Guilford Press.

Blackburn, R. (1993). *The psychology of criminal conduct: Theory, research and practice*. Chichester, England: John Wiley.

Bornstein, R. F. (1993). *The dependent personality*. New York: Guilford Press.

Clarkin, J. F. & Lenzenweger, M. E. (Eds.). (1996). *Major theories of personality disorder*. New York: Guilford Press.

Clarkin, J. F., Marziali, E. & Munroe-Blum, H. (Eds.). (1992). *Borderline personality disorder: Clinical and empirical perspectives*. New York: Guilford Press.

Cleckley, H. (1964). *The mask of sanity*. (4th edn). Saint Lousis, MO: Mosby.

Collins, S. & Cattermole, R. (2004). *Anti-Social behaviour: Power and remedies*. London: Sweet and Maxwell.

Cooke, D. J., Forth, A. E., & Hare, R. D. (Eds.). (1998). *Psychopathy: Theory, research, and implications for society*. Dordrecht, The Netherlands: Kluwer.

Costa, P. T. Jr. & Widiger, T. A. (Eds.). (1994). *Personality disorders and the five-factor model of personality*. Washington, DC: American Psychological Association.

Dawson, D. & MacMillan, H. L. (1993). *Relationship management of the borderline patient: From understanding to treatment*. New York: Brunner/Mazel.

Gunderson, J. G. (2001). *Borderline personality disorder: A clinical guide*. Washington, D.C: American Psychiatric Press.

Guntrip, H. (1969). *Schizoid phenomena, object relations and the self*. New York: International Universities Press.

Hare, R. D. (1993). *Without conscience: The disturbing world of the psychopaths among us*. New York: Simon and Schuster.

Horowitz, M. J. (Ed.). (1991). *Hysterical personality style and the histrionic personality disorder*. Northvale, NJ: Jason Aronson.

Kernberg, O. F. (1984). *Severe personality disorders*. New Haven: Yale University Press.

Lenzenweger, M. F. (2005). *Major theories of personality disorders*. New York: Guilford Press.

Linehan, M. M. (1993). *Cognitive behavioral therapy for borderline personality disorder*. New York: Guilford Press.

Livesley, J. (Ed.). (1995). *The DSM-IV personality disorders*. Washington, DC: American Psychiatric Association.

Livesley, W. J. (2001). *Handbook of personality disorders*. New York: Guilford Press.

Lykken, D. T. (1995). *The antisocial personalities*. Hillsdale, NJ: Erlbaum.

Maj, M., Akiskal, H. S., Mezzich, J. E., & Okasha, A. (Eds.). (2005). *Personality disorders*. New York: John Wiley and Sons.

Millon, T. & Davis, R. D. (1996). *Disorders of personality: DSM-IV and beyond*. New York: Wiley-Interscience.

Raine, A., Lencz, T., & Mednick, S. (Eds.). (1995). *Schizotypal personality*. New York: Cambridge University Press.

Ronningstam, E. (Ed.). (1998). *Disorders of narcissism: Diagnostic, clinical, and empirical implications*. Washington, DC: American Psychiatric Press.

Salzman, L. (1980). *Treatment of the obsessive personality*. New York: Jason Aronson.

Shapiro, D. (1965). *Neurotic styles*. New York: Basic Books.

Stoff, D. M., Maser, J., & Brieling, J. (Eds.). (1997). *Handbook of antisocial behaviour*. New York: John Wiley.

CHAPTER 9

The Substance Use Disorders

First Responders and law enforcement personnel are more likely to encounter individuals suffering from substance intoxication, abuse and/or dependence than any other psychiatric impairment. Use of all psychoactive substances in this country, including caffeine and nicotine, has a staggering impact on our economy, on the health of our citizens, and on the incidence of crime, violence, and homelessness in our cities. Statistics from the Bureau of Justice as well as several research studies indicate that alcohol and illicit drug users report increased criminal involvement, criminal records, and crime related violence than non-users. In an article entitled "Psychoactive Substances and Violence," published in 1994 by The Institute of Justice in its journal, *Research in Brief*, Jeffrey Roth notes that in recent years alcohol use by the perpetrator and/or the victim of a crime immediately preceded at least 50% of all violent episodes studied. Additionally, research he cites indicates that chronic drinkers and drug users are more likely to have histories of violence, and more likely to commit assaults and robberies, than non-users as well as criminals who do not use drugs or alcohol. There is no doubt that there is a strong relationship among violence, criminality, and use of psychoactive substances, and for this reason alone, understanding the nature of addiction and the common effects of drugs and alcohol is critical for First Responders. This chapter will review the major psychoactive substances, their principal effects on individuals, the nature of addiction, strategies for treatment, and the complex relationship between specific substances and violent and criminal behavior.

DIMENSIONS OF SUBSTANCE USE

A psychoactive substance is a chemical that, when ingested, alters brain function, specifically impacting perception, mood, consciousness, or behavior. Not all of these substances, however, are illegal or result in serious impairments in consciousness or violent behavior. Caffeine and nicotine are two examples that are used extensively throughout the world, can be very addictive, but typically involve the medical community rather than law enforcement personnel. The toll in health related problems for these substances is astronomical. The focus of this chapter, however, will be on those substances that are illegal and/or significantly alter psychological functions and behavior.

In order to begin to understand these serious substance related disorders, it is important to clarify the differences among several terms that have been used inappropriately at times to describe the problem. *Substance use* is a term that simply reflects the fact that an individual has used any substance in a moderate amount and only to the extent that the use does not impair daily functioning. An occasional cigarette, morning coffee, or a glass of wine with dinner represents common uses of psychoactive substances that are often part of daily life. When using a substance results in temporary maladaptive behavioral or psychological alterations in functioning such as dramatic mood changes, impairment in cognition and judgment, or aggression, the reaction is termed *substance intoxication*. The manifestations of intoxication will vary depending on the specific substance that is ingested. *Substance abuse* is defined by the DSM-IV-TR as a maladaptive pattern of substance use that results in the failure to function adequately in our important daily roles including work and school, frequently involving use in dangerous situations like driving, resulting in legal problems and continuing in spite of recurrent social and interpersonal problems. Finally, *substance dependence* is defined by the DSM-IV-TR as a maladaptive pattern of substance use that results in tolerance and withdrawal, in the tendency to use more drug than intended, in unsuccessful efforts to quit or cut down, in spending significant time trying to obtain the substance, in sacrifice of most normal activities as a result of drug use, and in the continued use of the substance in spite of recurrent physical and psychological problems related to its use. *Tolerance* refers to the individual's need for significantly more of the substance to produce the desired effect, while *withdrawal* refers to the distressing physiological and psychological consequences that are experienced when no longer taking the drug. Substance dependence has also been referred to as *addiction*.

Each psychoactive substance has a unique profile in terms of its effects on the central nervous system, in terms of the clinical picture of intoxication and withdrawal syndromes, its progression, as well as in terms of its contribution to violence and aggression. Five categories of psychoactive substances will be discussed in this chapter including depressants, stimulants, opiates, hallucinogens and other abused drugs.

DEPRESSANTS

Depressants are a class of substances, including alcohol, sedative, hypnotic and anxiolytic drugs, that basically reduce physiological arousal, help us feel less anxious, as well as allow us to relax and sleep.

Alcohol

Alcohol, or ethanol, is a highly addictive CNS depressant that is the most commonly used drug in the world. Produced by the action of yeast on carbohydrates in fruits and grains, beer, wine and liquor are consumed by nearly 50% of Americans over 12 years old. According to the American Council for Drug Addiction, there are up to 15 million alcoholics or problem drinkers in the United States and more than 100,000 deaths due to alcohol each year.

Alcohol has a paradoxical effect on our nervous system initially by acting as a stimulant allowing most users to feel relaxed, uninhibited, and often very social and extroverted. This occurs because alcohol affects the inhibitory mechanism in the brain. As more and more alcohol is consumed, the individual begins to experience increasing levels of cognitive confusion, impaired judgment, motor incoordination, sensory impairments like blurred vision and, in some cases, violent behavior. Five drinks (i.e. about 7.5 ounces of liquor) consumed in two hours may raise blood level to 0.10%, legally intoxicated in every state.

Chronic alcohol abuse and dependence may result in a variety of very severe psychiatric and medical conditions. Alcohol-induced persisting dementia and Wernicke's disease result in loss of intellectual abilities including abstract thinking and memory, as well as confusion and lack of muscle coordination. Many of these losses may be irreversible. Medical problems include cardiac disease, damage to the liver, pancreas, and kidneys, as well as serious impairments to pregnant women who may give birth to infants with significant developmental problems including fetal alcohol syndrome, described in Chapter Twelve. Withdrawal from chronic alcohol use can be a very dangerous and, at times, fatal syndrome. Alcohol withdrawal delirium, commonly known as the DT's or delirium tremens, results in tremors, agitation, anxiety, visual hallucinations, convulsions, and seizures. If not medically managed, it can result in death.

Alcohol is the only psychoactive substance that tends to increase aggressive and violent behavior temporarily in many individuals while they are using the substance. This is not to suggest that alcohol *causes* violence since several other factors may contribute to this relationship, including the users' pre-morbid personality, their history of violence, the settings in which they drink, and their expectations about drinking. There is no question that alcohol will increase the probability that the individuals will become more impulsive when they drink excessively and will gradually experience impaired judgment. In a study published in 1990 by Wieczorek and his colleagues in the *Journal of Criminal Justice*, results indicated that alcohol was directly implicated in nearly 50% of all homicides committed by nearly 2,000 homicide offenders whom they studied.

Sedative, Hypnotic, and Anxiolytic Substances

This group of depressant, psychoactive drugs produces calmness, sleep, and relaxation by affecting the same neurosynaptic pathways in the brain as alcohol. Often these sedative-hypnotic-anxiolytic drugs are referred to as tranquilizers and sleeping pills or, sometimes, just as sedatives. *Barbiturates* and *benzodiazepines* are the two major categories of sedative-hypnotics. Common barbiturates include Seconal, Nembutal, and Amytal. Valium, Librium, Xanax, and Tranxene are examples of benzodiazepines that are commonly used and abused today.

Barbiturates have been used in the past by physicians for sleep, but in recent years have been a major drug of abuse with relatively few legitimate medical uses. Barbiturates are often called "barbs" and "downers." The effects of these drugs are similar to those of alcohol, with small amounts producing calmness and relaxation, and increased dosages resulting in slurred speech, staggering gait, and poor judgment. Overdoses often occur when barbiturates are combined with alcohol, or when a user takes one dose, becomes confused, and unintentionally takes additional doses. The dose required for the "therapeutic" or desired mental state and the toxic dose of barbiturates are very close together. In sum, barbiturate overdose is a factor in nearly one-third of all reported drug-related deaths according to the National Institute of Drug Abuse. Benzodiazepines are often used therapeutically to reduce anxiety in psychiatric and other medical patients, but in recent years have also become abused street drugs. As an odorless substitute for alcohol, many teenagers have begun to abuse these drugs. Rohypnol or "roofies" are in this class of drugs which have become known as the "date rape" drug. Men have placed the drug in the drinks of unsuspecting women whose defenses and inhibitions are compromised and later sexually assaulted them.

Benzodiazepines, like alcohol, can cause both psychological and physical dependence, as well as the development of tolerance over time. Abruptly discontinuing barbiturates and benzodiazepines often may result in withdrawal symptoms including restlessness, anxiety, convulsions, and even death.

STIMULANTS

Stimulants encompass groups of drugs that increase energy, alertness and physical activity, and include amphetamines and cocaine as well as the commonly used nicotine and caffeine.

Amphetamines

Amphetamines, like Ritalin, are prescribed by physicians for specific disorders and are often used in appropriate doses to treat narcolepsy as well as attention deficit hyperactivity disorder in both children and adults. Amphetamines increase heart rate, dilate the pupils, increase blood pressure, and decrease appetite. As the dose increases, individuals often experience anxiety, anger, poor judgment, chills, nausea, psychomotor agitation, or retardation, cardiac arrhythmias, confusion, convulsion, and coma. While the users may initially feel full of energy and confidence, abuse may lead to repetitive, stereotyped behaviors, and psychotic behavior, including hallucinations, delusions, and paranoia. At first glance, patients displaying these symptoms may be seen as suffering from a schizophrenic disorder whose active phase appears very similar.

Amphetamines, commonly referred to as "speed" or "uppers," are psychologically addictive and can lead to the need for larger doses and/or the use of cocaine. Abrupt termination can result in fatigue, irritability, depression or "crashing," and fatigue. An amphetamine commonly called "Ecstasy" has become a popular designer drug often used in the "club scene," it is noted for enhancing the users' feelings of euphoria. Methamphetamine, referred to as "crystal meth" or "ice," has become epidemic in some areas of the country and with specific groups. It is manufactured cheaply in home laboratories and has become a major problem for law enforcement personnel since it increases the possibility of aggressive and violent behavior in users (Table 9.1).

Cocaine

Cocaine has emerged as a major abused drug since the early 1970s and has gained notoriety given its popularity with the rich and famous, and as a result of the crime and violence that has been associated with its illegal sale. Widely used in the past as an ingredient in many different patent medicines developed to treat hunger, fatigue, and concentration problems, up until 1903, it was used even in Coca-Cola. Pure cocaine is a white powder derived from the leaves of the coca plant common in South America. Typically, it is inhaled through the nose where it can be absorbed quickly, but it can also be liquefied and inhaled with a pipe in a ritual called "freebasing." A form of cocaine called "crack" or "rock" cocaine is used in this way. Freebasing using crack cocaine introduces a very high concentration of the drug into the bloodstream very quickly, and its use can be very dangerous and very highly addictive.

Similar to amphetamines, cocaine produces feelings of euphoria, a "rush" and a sense of having more energy and power. However, these initial feelings wear off quickly, and the user must ingest more cocaine to prevent "crashing" and ultimately feeling depressed. Additionally,

Table 9.1. Consequences of Methamphetamine Abuse

- Sleeplessness
- Loss of appetite
- Elevated body temperature
- Paranoia
- Depression and anxiety
- Seizures
- Permanent damage to brain cells

Table 9.2. Consequences of Cocaine and Crack Abuse

- Cardiovascular problems
- Stroke, seizures and brain infections
- Lung disorders
- Psychosis
- Sexual dysfunction
- Increased risk of traumatic injury from accidents and criminal behavior

users will experience increased heart rate, increased blood pressure, agitation, and cardiac problems. Over time, many individuals will experience feelings of paranoia and will ultimately manifest impairments in concentration, memory, and overall daily functioning. In contrast to alcohol withdrawal, cocaine withdrawal results in apathy, boredom, and feelings of depression (Table 9.2).

OPIOIDS

Opioids refer to a family of drugs that encompass the natural opiates including opium, morphine, heroin, codeine, and synthetic varieties including methadone. It also includes natural brain chemicals like endorphins that are activated by these drugs and result in the "rush" sought after by the abusers. Opium derived from the opium poppy is a dark brown sticky resin which is commonly smoked or eaten. Heroin is a white or brownish powder that is usually dissolved in water and then injected, or even smoked. Opiates and their derivatives have an important medical application, especially in the reduction of pain, but have a high potential for abuse and dependence. Typically, they are liquefied and injected, producing feelings of relaxation, euphoria, and reduction of anxiety. Intoxication will also involve feelings of apathy, depression, psychomotor retardation, impaired judgment, pupillary constriction, impaired memory, and concentration. Opiate overdose can lead to impairments in respiration and ultimately death.

Heroin

The opiate heroin does not have many legal medical applications today and has been replaced by synthetic analgesics. Heroin is snorted, injected, inhaled or swallowed by the user, and is often mixed by street dealers with other substances to reduce its potency. Tolerance builds up over time and may require that the abuser "shoot up" several times a day to maintain the "high." Besides the risk of heroin overdose resulting in respiratory failure and death, the method of ingestion will often represent a major health risk for the user. Contaminated needles risk blood infections, infection from the HIV virus, and Hepatitis B and C.

Table 9.3. Consequences of Heroin Use

- Loss of appetite, nausea
- Menstrual irregularity
- Reduced sex drive
- Fatigue, labored breathing
- Hepatitis, AIDS
- Stroke or heart attack
- Coma, Death from overdose

Dependence, both physiological and psychological, will inevitably occur over time. Withdrawal is often quite severe, with symptoms of nausea, insomnia, diarrhea, anxiety and tremors lasting a few days. The life of a heroin addict is likely to be relatively short, many dying of overdose, homicide, suicide, or accident by middle age (Table 9.3).

Synthetic Opioids

Methadone is a synthetic narcotic, sometimes used medically to reduce pain, but more typically given as a legal, therapeutic, and more medically safe substitute for heroin. It blocks the effects of heroin and reduces physical cravings. When given in appropriate dosages, it produces mild euphoria and sedation, while eliminating the risk of respiratory failure more common with heroin. When given as part of a therapeutic drug maintenance program, it eliminates addicts' search for illegal heroin, eliminates the use of needles since it is administered orally, but, unfortunately, continues to insure that the user remains addicted to an opioid. Methadone withdrawal, however, is much less severe than that of heroin.

Semisynthetic Derivatives

Today, one of the most abused prescription opioids is oxycodone, a very potent and addictive pain killer that is marketed as Percodan, Percocet or OxyContin. Medically indicated for severe pain on a short-term basis, more extended use and abuse will result in tolerance and dependence. Unlike Percodan and Percocet that combine oxycodone with aspirin or acetaminophen, respectively, OxyContin is pure oxycodone. Abusers can crush the tablets, and snort or inject the resulting powder to achieve rapid absorption into the bloodstream and an immediate "high." The illegal sale and abuse of these drugs has posed a major problem for law enforcement personnel in the past five years.

HALLUCINOGENS

Hallucinogens are substances, both natural and synthetic, that significantly alter users' perceptions, sensations, emotions, and cognitions. Natural hallucinogens include mescaline that comes from the peyote cactus; marijuana, from the hemp plant; and psilocybin derived from mushrooms. Synthetic drugs include Ecstacy and PCP, while LSD is considered semisynthetic since it is derived from a fungus growing on rye grains, but is subject to considerable chemical processing. The DSM-IV-TR characterizes hallucinogen intoxication as involving significant behavioral and psychological changes causing anxiety and depression, fear of losing one's mind, and impaired functioning, all accompanied by perceptual changes that occur while the individual is fully awake and alert, including depersonalization, derealization, hallucinations, and illusions. Additionally, users will manifest other symptoms including pupillary dilation, rapid heartbeat, blurred vision, and motor incoordination. Different users will experience different effects with these drugs based on the amount taken, their personality and expectations, as well as their environment at the time. Some hallucinogens create sensations and feelings that are often labile, constantly changing, at times seeming to "cross over." Users will report that they "hear" colors and "see" sounds. Some of these perceptual changes are quite frightening; they may result in feelings of confusion and loss of control, and may even precipitate a psychotic reaction in a predisposed individual.

Marijuana

Marijuana is the most commonly used illegal drug today. Cannabis, its formal name, is derived from the hemp plant whose psychoactive ingredient is delta-9-tetrahydrocannabinol (THC). The THC content of marijuana has changed drastically over the past thirty years, creating a much more potent drug today that is typically smoked in a rolled cigarette or "joint," brewed into tea, or baked in cookies or brownies. Moderate amounts of marijuana or "pot" create a feeling of euphoria, relaxation and, like other hallucinogens, alterations in perception. Additionally, users will experience motor incoordination, sensation of slowed time, social withdrawal, increased appetite, dry mouth and rapid heart rate. High dosages can result in paranoia and hallucinations in some individuals. Over time, research has shown that chronic use leads to cognitive problems including impairments in concentration, memory, and attention, as well as in the loss of motivation for productive activity (Table 9.4).

Table 9.4. Consequences of Marijuana Abuse

- Impaired perception
- Diminished short term memory
- Loss of concentration
- Loss of motivation
- Anxiety and paranoia
- Psychological dependence

Table 9.5. Consequences of LSD Abuse

- High temperature
- Increased blood pressure
- Sleeplessness
- Appetite loss
- Tremors
- Flashbacks

LSD

LSD is the most common and best known hallucinogen. It is generally ingested orally in small dosages and comes in squares on sheets, like postage stamps, in small "microdots," or gelatin squares, or in liquid form dispensed with an eyedropper. Users experience alterations in perception, distorting time, space, and distance, as well as creating vivid visual hallucinations of color and "psychedelic" patterns. LSD often distorts judgment and causes anxiety, panic, and psychotic behavior in a "bad trip." *Flashbacks* often occur involving the reoccurrence of the LSD experience, sometimes days or months after the actual ingestion and without any additional drug (Table 9.5).

OTHER ABUSED DRUGS

PCP, Ecstasy, Ketamine, and GHB

PCP or "angel dust," initially developed as an anesthetic in the late 1950s, is a white, crystalline powder, produced in illegal labs and usually smoked, snorted or injected. The effects, like many of the other drugs described above, are variable, with moderate doses producing relaxation, euphoria, feelings of power, and dissociated, or "spaced out" experiences. Physically, users experience rapid heart rate, increased body temperature, numbness and incoordination. As doses increase, there is greater likelihood of nausea, mood swings, aggressiveness, and violence, and, when mixed with other drugs, convulsions and death. PCP can often precipitate psychotic episodes, particularly in individuals with pre-existing psychiatric illness. A related drug, ketamine, is a powdery substance that is typically snorted or smoked, and produces hallucinations, a sense of detachment, and reduction of pain.

Ecstasy is a synthetic hallucinogenic stimulant whose effects are similar to those of amphetamines and hallucinogens. Illegal like heroin, cocaine and LSD, Ecstasy acts as a mood enhancer inducing feelings of euphoria, relaxation, and, reportedly, feelings of love, insight, and deep understanding of others. It has gained popularity with young people who enjoy the "club scene," and dance parties called "raves" where they dance for hours without stopping. Overdose of this drug results in high body temperature (hyperthermia), which is exacerbated by excessive physical activity, over stimulation of the nervous and cardiac systems, psychosis, respiratory symptoms, and possible death. GHB, sometimes called liquid Ecstasy, is a central nervous system depressant that produces a state of relaxation and talkativeness in lower doses, but, especially in combination with alcohol or other drugs, can result in seizures and coma. It was originally used by body builders to build muscles and was sold in health food stores, but was later banned by the Food and Drug Administration because of the severe side effects.

Steroids

Anabolic steroids are powerful drugs that historically have been taken in high doses by professional athletes in order to boost their performance. They help build muscle tissue and increase body mass by simulating the body's natural male hormone, testosterone. Anabolic steroids have been referred to as "roids," "juice," "hype," or "pump." Lower doses of these steroids sometimes are used to treat a few serious medical conditions. They should not be confused with *corticosteroids*, which are used to treat common medical conditions such as asthma and arthritis. Corticosteroids do not have muscle-building effects. While athletes primarily have been associated with steroid use and have gained recent notoriety in scandals associated with professional baseball, the reality, however, is that individuals pursuing the perfect, muscular body have been the fastest-growing group of steroid users in the United States.

The physical effects of steroid abuse can be serious and life threatening. Immediate effects in men can include shrinking of the testes and severe acne. Since anabolic steroids boost testosterone levels, women manifest their effects by becoming "virilized," including the deepening of their voices, irregular or nonexistent menses, male-pattern baldness, and sterility. Other physical effects for both sexes include hypertension, liver damage, stroke, and sleep disturbance. Emotional consequences include severe aggressive behavior, known as "roid rage," mood swings, hallucinations, paranoia, anxiety, and depression.

Inhalants

Inhalants are substances that produce a very quick and cheap high, resulting initially in lightheadedness and mild euphoria and later by drowsiness, headache, nausea, incoordination, and slurred speech. Many household products can be abused including organic solvents like gasoline, lighter fluid, nail polish remover, and airplane glue; nitrites that relax the blood vessels including amyl nitrite that is stored in glass capsules often referred to as "poppers" when they are broken; and nitrous oxide, known as "laughing gas," that produces a pleasant, altered state of consciousness that dentists use to reduce the perception of pain. Most often solvents are inhaled by spraying them on a piece of cloth or placing them in a plastic bag and placing the bag over a user's mouth and nose.

Inhalants are quite dangerous, potentially causing respiratory depression, coma and death. In heavy doses, they result in confusion, psychotic behavior including hallucinations and paranoid delusions. Long term use risks permanent brain damage as well as fatal damage to the liver and kidneys, the heart and CNS (Table 9.6).

Table 9.7 lists the street names for many of the drugs discussed below.

Table 9.6. Consequences of Inhalant Abuse

- Permanent brain damage
- Poor memory
- Extreme mood swings
- Tremors
- Seizures
- Cardiac arrhythmia
- Fatal damage to liver and kidneys

Table 9.7. Street Names for Common Drugs

Drug	Street names
Heroin	Smack, horse, H, junk, scag, blows, Charley, witch hazel
OxyContin	Oxy, OxyCotton, Oxy 80, OC, hillbilly heroin
Powder Cocaine	All American drug, big C, blow, nose candy, Florida snow
Crack Cocaine	Black rock, CD's, purple caps, soup, twinkie
Methamphetamine	Speed, meth, crank, crystal-meth, glass, blade, chrome, trash
Marijuana	Aunt Mary, blue sage, doobee, ganga, mary jane, weed
LSD	Acid, blue barrels, dots, sunshine, loony tunes
PCP	Wet, bobbies, dippies, dank, amp, hydro, haze, lillie, angel dust
Ecstasy	E, Adam, Roll, Bean, X, XTC, clarity, Stacy, Lover's speed
Inhalants	Air blasts, high ball, hippie crack, Texas shoe shine, moon gas
Ketamine	Cat valium, jet, purple, Special K,
Rohypnol	Forget pill, lunch money drug, R-2, roofies
Barbiturates	Barbs, downers, goofballs, sopers, luds
GHB	Fantasy, G, liquid G, Vita-G, jib, Georgia home boy

THE ETIOLOGY OF SUBSTANCE ABUSE
AND DEPENDENCE

The causes of substance abuse and dependence have been a source of considerable controversy and confusion as well as an area of considerable research over the years. The lay public, politicians, the medical community, and law enforcement personnel have struggled to unravel those factors that lead individuals to use, abuse and, ultimately, to become dependent on psychoactive substances. Some have endorsed a *moral weakness* model of etiology that asserts that drug use is the result of a failure of self control and character strength that makes it difficult for an individual to "Say no to drugs." Such a philosophy has led to condemnation and, frequently, to punishment as a way to address the problem. Others have embraced a *disease model* of etiology based on the notion that substance abuse and dependence arise from underlying biological deficits that influence and/or determine individuals' unique reaction to psychoactive drugs. Obviously, this perspective has informed a treatment and rehabilitation oriented approach to abuse and addiction. Neither of these very different models can explain the complex problem of drug use and, like many of the other psychological disorders described in these chapters, researchers and clinicians must look to the interplay of biological, psychosocial, and cultural factors in order to begin to unravel the causes.

Genetics have been found to play a critical role in the development of several disorders we have discussed, including schizophrenia and the mood disorders. Research in the area of substance abuse has found that certain individuals may have a genetic predisposition to drug abuse in general and alcohol abuse in particular. Family, adoption, and twin studies suggest that a history of alcohol abuse and dependence in one's biological relatives will determine to some extent the risk of alcohol problems in their offspring, particularly in men. The mode of inheritance is not clear, nor have specific genes been identified conclusively. Research by Kendler and his colleagues in a 2003 study published in the *Journal of Psychiatry* studied over 1,000 pairs of twins and inquired about their use of several types of drugs from opiates to stimulants. Results indicated that genetic influences seemed to impact all drug use. The use of illicit drugs, however, was impacted primarily by psychosocial factors, while abuse and dependence may be the end result of some genetic predisposition. Environment, it would seem, plays a major role in determining whether or not individuals use these illegal substances, but biology becomes dominant in determining the likelihood of addiction.

In the simplest terms, psychoactive drug users and abusers will acknowledge that their primary motivation for using drugs is to "feel good" and to avoid "feeling bad." The biological substrate for this effect lies in the reward centers in the brain where the drugs like cocaine, heroin, and amphetamines seem to impact on the availability of neurotransmitters, in particular, dopamine. Alcohol and the benzodiazepines help individuals avoid pain by reducing anxiety, a mechanism involving the GABA neuroreceptor system in the brain.

Another model of etiology of substance use and abuse involves the basic principles of learning theory. The pleasurable and "feel good" experiences of psychoactive drugs act as a *positive reinforcer* for this behavior that will increase the likelihood of continued use and eventually the possibility of tolerance and dependence The concept of *negative reinforcement* explains how the user will avoid distressing feelings by ingesting drugs that reduce anxiety, physical pain and feelings of insecurity. Continued abuse is reinforced when the initial "high" is followed by the unpleasant withdrawal. To avoid this pain, the user must ingest more of the drug. Alcohol abusers deal with their "hangover" by drinking more alcohol or having "the hair of the dog that bite[s them]."

Individuals suffering from the debilitating effects of medical as well as psychiatric illness are prescribed psychoactive drugs legally to relieve pain and the symptoms of anxiety and depression. Many of these potential medical and psychiatric patients, however, may not seek out appropriate professional care, but rather medicate themselves with drugs like cocaine or oxycontin that may initially relieve physical or psychic pain, but eventually lead to addiction and sometimes death. While such individuals had suffered initially from a single medical or psychological disorder, their decision to medicate themselves may soon leave them with a new problem, a substance abuse disorder. Individuals with schizophrenia, depression, post traumatic stress, and physical pain disorders are particularly vulnerable to this problem. Law enforcement personnel struggle with the homeless populations in their communities, where most of these individuals have psychiatric problems complicated by significant substance abuse involvement.

Social and cultural factors also play a role in the use and abuse of all psychoactive substances. The reader needs only to turn on the television or read popular magazines to understand how our society reinforces the notion that it is important to feel good, avoid discomfort and turn to medication to accomplish these goals. Social modeling of parents as well as peers will have an impact on how children and adolescents perceive drug use. Research confirms that alcoholism runs in families and that some of the influences result from environmental factors in addition to biology. Different cultures and religions deal with substance use in unique ways. For instance, Jewish culture frowns on intoxication in any context, while some Asian cultures encourage heavy alcohol use in certain social situations. In all likelihood, culture and genetics interact in producing the unique patterns of use, abuse, and dependence seen in each cultural group. Box 9.1 addresses the relationship between drug addiction and our biological makeup.

BOX 9.1
Brain Studies and Drug Addiction

Wired, but why? Studies of cells in the brain may explain why some people are more likely than others to become hooked on drugs.

By Douglas Birch
Baltimore Sun reporter
February 24, 2006

It wrecks neighborhoods, families and lives, and might be the most important public health problem faced by Western societies. Yet since chemists first isolated cocaine, morphine and heroin in the 19th century, physicians and scientists have struggled to explain the nature of addiction.

There is still much to learn, but with advances in genetics, medical imaging technology and neuroscience, scientists say they are closer than ever to understanding why some people who try drugs become addicted, and some do not.

"I think we made more progress in the last 10 years than in the previous history of mankind," said Frank Vocci, director of treatment and research at the National Institute on Drug Abuse, which spends $1 billion annually on drug research.

"We're a heck of a lot further along than we were 30 years ago," said Dr. Paul R. McHugh, a psychiatrist at the Johns Hopkins School of Medicine. That progress, he added, "tells me that we don't have to be quite as hopeless as we were before about addicts."

In the past decade, scientists have come to recognize that genetics plays a major role in all addictions. It was long suspected that alcoholism was at least partly inherited because of its presence in some families and not others. But studies of addicts in Baltimore, Japan and elsewhere have shown that methamphetamine users, heroin addicts and other habitual drug users share similar variants of dozens of brain receptor genes.

One day, scientists say, genetic testing could enable drug counselors to warn parents if their children carry an unusually high risk of addiction, or tailor existing treatments to individual drug users. But the ultimate hope, of course, is that the genetics of addiction will help find powerful new treatments. So far, the development of new addiction treatments has lagged far behind the basic science. "There have been modest, incremental improvements," said Dr. Solomon H. Snyder, a Johns Hopkins neuroscientist and psychiatrist who is one of the world's authorities on the biochemistry of addiction. In general, he said, advances have come slowly because major pharmaceutical companies see little profit in tackling the problem. But by defining what addiction is, researchers have helped the pharmaceutical industry identify what it calls "targets" for drug research—genes, proteins, neurotransmitters that could be modified to block the compulsive use of drugs. One thing that addiction is not, scientists say, is a simple inherited illness. There is no single gene that inevitably leads to habitual drug use. Instead, some people appear to carry an array of genes that raises their risk of addiction.

"Nobody has to become addicted," said Dr. George R. Uhl, a clinical neurologist and chief of the National Institute on Drug Abuse's molecular neurobiology branch at Hopkins' Bayview campus.

"Genes have an influence on behavior," McHugh said. "They're not a determining influence on behavior, in that if you've got them there's nothing you can do about them. They are an influence."

Overall, researchers say, about half of an individual's susceptibility to addiction is inherited, while the other half is the product of a person's environment—which includes the pressures of family, peers and neighborhood.

Discussions of addiction usually focus on people living in the most desperate circumstances, in the poorest neighborhoods. But the problem, of course, extends far beyond the inner city.

Lee Krol was a skilled marine electrician, homeowner and father who lived in Pasadena. But he had a problem that anguished and mystified his family for most of his life. As a teenager, he began to drink and use drugs. While he would quit for a while, it was never for good. "There's nothing like this stuff," he once told his brother, Tom.

So his family was devastated, but not surprised, when they found the 50-year-old on the floor of the computer room of his home December 7, dead of a heroin overdose. "I want him to be portrayed as a good person," said Tom Krol. "He just had a terrible disease."

Since the early 1970s, scientists have identified all of the brain cell switches, called receptors, which respond to addictive drugs. Using advanced imaging technology such as MRI machines and PET scanners, they have been able to watch as drugs alter the way the biochemical signals called thoughts and feelings are transmitted through the brain. Addiction research has zeroed in on a group of brain cells in the nucleus accumbens, nestled deep within the brain, the location of what has been called the "pleasure reward" system. Many of the brain cells, or neurons, in this network communicate with each other with two of the brain's chemical messengers, serotonin and dopamine.

The system produces feelings of well being, the reward for engaging in actions such as eating and sex, vital to survival and reproduction. Illicit drugs, it turns out, switch on this system—specifically, by raising the level of dopamine available to neurons. Dopamine receptors, scientists say, appear to play an important role in all three of the main features of addiction—tolerance, withdrawal and compulsive drug seeking.

Despite the recent advances in the lab, much of the way this system works remains a mystery, Snyder said. Recent research, though, offers some clues.

Using advanced imaging technology, scientists have discovered that people whose brains have a higher concentration of the so-called D2 dopamine receptor reacted with indifference to a mild stimulant—in this case, Ritalin—while those with fewer D2 receptors tended to enjoy the experience. Dr. Nora Volkow, one of the nation's leading addiction researchers and director of NIDA, led studies showing that cocaine users have lower concentrations of D2 receptors than nonusers.

It's not clear whether people are born with higher D2 receptor densities, develop higher densities as a result of experience, or both. In a paper in the journal Nature Neuroscience in 2002, scientists at Wake Forest University showed that macaque monkeys that achieve high status in small groups tend to develop a higher concentration of D2 receptors. The D2 density of subordinate macaques did not change.

This work suggests that there is a link between low status, D2 density and vulnerability to addiction. But this picture may not be as simple as it seems, said Snyder, who helped launch modern addiction research in 1973, when he and his student, Candace Pert, discovered the opiate receptor. When researchers in his lab exposed rodents to mind-altering drugs, Snyder said, they would typically find that hundreds of genes in the rodents became more active—raising, say, the number of receptors—and hundreds became less active.

"From our experience with rodents, D2 receptors went up, but probably another 299 things went up, too," he said. Tracking a single change in a single receptor does not establish a cause-and-effect relationship. Still, some scientists say that advances in genetics research could have practical applications. Uhl, the NIDA neurologist at Bayview, points out that Naltrexone, used to block the effects of alcohol, works better for people with one form of a gene than another.

"If you have a genetic test that tells you the drug is twice as likely to be effective in this person than that one, you could focus the treatment in ways that are the most likely to have benefits," Uhl said. "That seems like a huge potential positive impact."

Drugs developed to treat other diseases are being used to help addicts. Smokers are often given anti-depressants, for example, to help them overcome their dependence on nicotine—which ranks with cocaine as the most powerfully addictive of the widely used drugs (Without treatment, only one out of 20 smokers quits successfully, researchers say).

One of the most successful treatments for habitual drug users, said Michael Gimbel, a former heroin addict and director of substance abuse at Sheppard Pratt Health System in Towson, are Alcoholics Anonymous-style "12-step" programs, in which addicts guaranteed anonymity encourage one another to overcome their dependence.

Many drug users will need more intensive, residential treatment. Tom Krol said his brother, Lee, needed residential treatment, but could not afford to take the necessary time off from work.

The public, frustrated by the seeming intractability of addiction, is reluctant to pay for expensive treatment programs, researchers point out. As a result, there is a chronic shortage of spaces or "slots" in such programs nationwide. Snyder of Hopkins said that Maryland's General Assembly is considering a bill to spend $125 million over five years on stem cell research. Why, he asked, aren't legislators seeking a similar crash program to develop new treatments for drug abuse? Curbing addiction would have direct relevance to one of the most important health challenges facing Baltimore and other Maryland communities. Such a program, he said, would have a better chance of success than many other research efforts, because so much of the groundwork has been laid.

The prospect of new stem cell treatments "is a way-, way-, way-off hope," Snyder said. "If we did something about drug addiction, if we had research focused on therapies, there we would have a payoff in the much-nearer term."

TREATMENT OF SUBSTANCE ABUSE AND DEPENDENCE

Alcohol and drug abuse treatment is typically a multi-faceted program of education, counseling, and therapy that is commonly referred to as rehabilitation. Based on the philosophy that addiction is a disease rather than a moral weakness, "rehab" programs help individuals learn to control their disorder and lead productive and substance-free lives. The immediate goals of treatment are to reduce drug use, assist the patient in functioning more effectively without drugs, and to reduce the many complications of drug abuse including physical and legal problems. For most programs, the ultimate goal of treatment is to enable the addict to achieve lasting abstinence.

Alcohol and drug abuse rehabilitation programs are designed to meet the specific needs of the patient and are represented by several different delivery models. The most impaired and dependent users are typically referred to an inpatient residential program where detoxification is the first order of business. Detox is designed to treat the medical complications of withdrawal and minimize the distress individuals are likely to experience. After the individual is free of the substance, treatment often continues for 3 to 6 weeks comprising a combination of education and therapy during which the addict learns about alcohol and drug abuse dependency and how to work a program of recovery. Therapy generally consists of group, family, and individual counseling focusing on interpersonal functioning, spiritual issues, and stress management. With the advent of managed care and the pressure to reduce the high costs of treatment, many programs have eliminated all but inpatient detox and focused on the delivery of services in an outpatient setting.

Less restrictive and more cost effective approaches involve partial hospitalization programs where individuals return to their homes each night, intensive outpatient programs involving office visits, often after work in the evening, for three to five evenings a week, as well as traditional outpatient visits to an office or clinic on a weekly basis. All of these programs consist of substance abuse education; individual, family and group counseling; and, typically, a Twelve Step component based on the Alcoholics Anonymous program established in 1935. Offshoots of this program have evolved to cover most "addictions" including Narcotics Anonymous, Overeaters Anonymous, Sex Addicts Anonymous, and Gamblers Anonymous. All of these 12 Step models are predicated on a philosophy that asserts that an addict suffers from a disease over which they have no control. In order to recover, users must look to their "Higher Power," rely on the support of their social group and "work a program" dedicated to addressing personal and interpersonal flaws. By far, the Twelve Step program is the most common form of substance abuse treatment, in spite of the fact that it has little empirical research to support its efficacy. There is no question, however, that especially when combined with more traditional forms of treatment, Twelve Step programs increase the probability of recovery from alcoholism and drug abuse.

While psychosocial treatments are the most successful of the interventions designed to enable alcohol and substance abusers to maintain sobriety, there are some adjuctive biological treatments employed by physicians that are designed to counter or replace the addicting properties of alcohol and other drugs. One of the most popular interventions in the treatment of heroin addiction is the use of methadone. As discussed earlier, methadone is a synthetic narcotic that is legal and reduces the medical complications of heroin. The heroin user, however, is likely to become addicted to methadone since it affects the same neurosynaptic receptors in the brain. Another drug called naltrexone blocks the effects of the opiates and eliminates the euphoria associated with this class of drugs. It has very modest success with abusers who are not highly motivated and who are not participating in a comprehensive treatment program. Naltrexone has also been used in the treatment of alcoholism. In both cases, the drug may assist in blunting the effects of substance withdrawal and drug cravings, but alone is of little help in the recovery process. Finally, clinicians have used the drug Antabuse in the treatment of alcoholism. When individuals drink alcohol after taking Antabuse, they experience very aversive consequences including nausea, vomiting, rapid heart rate and respiration. This aversive experience will insure that abusers will avoid alcohol as long as they are taking the medication. However, unmotivated alcoholics will simply discontinue the drug and, after a few days, resume their drinking. Again, these biological interventions are no replacement for addicts' sincere motivation to change and a structured and comprehensive rehabilitation program.

SUGGESTED READINGS

Collins, R., Leonard, K., & Searles, J. (Eds.). (1990). *Alcohol and the family: Research and clinical perspectives*. New York: Guilford Press.

Donovan, D. M. & Marlatt, G. A. (Eds.). (1988). *Assessment of addictive behaviors*. New York: Guilford Press.

Galanter, M. (Ed.). (2003). *Recent developments in alcoholism*. Vol. 16. New York: Springer.

Galanter, M. & Kleber, H. D. (Eds.). (1994). *Textbook of substance abuse treatment*. Washington, DC: American Psychiatric Press.

Gislason, S. J. (2006). *The book of alcohol*. Environmental Research, Inc.

Gomberg, E. L. & Nirenberg, T. D. (Eds.). (1995). *Women and substance abuse*. Norwood, NJ: Ablex Publishing.

Horgan, C. (1993). *Substance Abuse: The Nation's number one health problem*. Princeton, NJ: Robert Wood Johnson Foundation.

Juhnke, G. A. (2002). *Substance abuse assessment and diagnosis: A comprehensive guide for counselors and helping professionals*. Routledge.

Leonard, K. E. & Blane, H. T. (Eds.). (1999). *Psychological theories of drinking and alcoholism*. New York: Guilford Press.

Maistro, S. A., Galizio, M., & Connors, G. J. (1995). *Drug use and abuse* (2nd edn). Fort Worth: Harcourt Press.

Ray, O. & Ksir, C. (1996). *Drugs, society, and human behavior*. (7th edn). St. Louis: Mosby-Year Book.

Rivers, P. C. (Ed.). (1987). *Alcohol and addictive behavior*. Lincoln, NE: University of Nebraska Press.

Rose, R. M. & Barnett, J. (Eds.). (1988). *Alcoholism: Origins and outcome*. New York: Raven Press.

Schuckit, M. A. (2000). *Drug and alcohol abuse: A clinical guide to diagnosis and treatment*. New York: Springer.

Sims, B. (2005). *Substance Abuse Treatment with Correctional Clients*. New York: Haworth Press.

Sloboda, Z. (2005). *Epidemiology of drug abuse*. New York: Springer.

Wagner, E. F. & Waldron, H. B. (Eds.). (2001). *Innovations in adolescent substance abuse interventions*. Oxford: Elsevier Press.

Wright, F. D., Beck, A. T., Newman, C. F., & Liese, B. S. (2001). *Cognitive therapy of substance abuse*. New York: Guilford Press.

Zernig, G., Saria, A., O'Malley, S. S., & Kurz, M. (Eds.). (2000). *Handbook of alcoholism*. New York: CRC Press.

CHAPTER 10

Crisis, Terrorism and Trauma-Based Disorders

When thoughts of a crisis arise, September 11, 2001 is a date that is emblazoned in the minds of most people around the world, especially Americans. That date is also contemporaneous with the start of the current War on Terrorism being led by the United States. It is not common for people to have experienced a violent collective trauma such as a war, or a natural disaster such as an earthquake, a tsunami, or a hurricane personally, although most of us have experienced these disasters second-hand by watching television. However, most people have experienced smaller crises in their lives, such as violence in their family. The devastation of the gulf coast of Mississippi, Alabama, and Louisiana and the total destruction of the city of New Orleans from hurricane Katrina in September of 2005 sent over 500,000 people fleeing for their lives across the entire United States. Just a few weeks later, Hurricane Rita caused another million people to leave Texas and the surrounding gulf areas, while the already crippled levees finally gave way and once again flooded many parts of New Orleans. Then, South Florida, already dealing with the aftermath of Katrina when it swept through there before going on to the gulf coast, experienced Hurricane Wilma, causing further destruction and fear. There has been a good deal of study into the psychological effects of these experiences on survivors, and comparisons have been made between those effects and the effects on those who have experienced more common traumas such as physical and sexual abuse in the family and between intimate partners.

The impact from these situational experiences can produce psychological problems that mimic or enhance more serious mental illnesses. Equally troubling to those First Responders who deal with crises on a regular basis is the secondary impact of crises and trauma on them after listening to many stories of survivors. From these accounts, we are developing a literature on resilience or the ability of some survivors to be able to turn the crisis situation into a positive growth experience despite the trauma they have experienced. Look at the recovery story of Trisha Meili, the woman who was beaten and raped and left to die in Central Park in New York City in Box 10.1.

BOX 10.1

Trisha Meili, The "Central Park Jogger"

*Excerpts from Story by Marilyn Elias
USA Today, June 29, 2005*

Trisha Meili, the "Central Park jogger," was given last rites after her rape and savage beating in New York 16 years ago, a crime that appalled people all over the USA. Only the soles of her feet were unbruised. Multiple gashes split Meili's scalp; an eye socket was fractured in 21 places. She could not breathe on her own, lost most of her blood and had severe brain damage.

Doctors doubted the 28-year-old investment banker would survive. One even told her parents, "It might be better for all if Trisha died."

But she didn't die. She awoke from a 12-day coma to an apparently shattered life. A Phi Beta Kappa with two graduate degrees from Yale, Meili had been on the fast track to a vice presidency at Salomon Brothers. Now she couldn't even walk, talk, read or button her own blouse.

Sixteen years later, this same woman drew a standing ovation after speeches to the American Psychiatric Association and the American Psychological Association Meetings on recovery from trauma.

Meili didn't just survive; she thrived and grew. Of course, she had excellent medical care. But why didn't she dive into a spiral of depression and fury over the damage done to her? Where did she find the gumption to keep "pushing the envelope" of the limits of brain recovery?

Mental health experts are paying more attention to robust survivors such as Meili in light of a rapidly growing "positive psychology" movement that focuses on how to build human strengths and happiness. Published studies on these topics have increased by about 60% in the past four years, says University of Pennsylvania psychologist Martin E.P. Seligman.

"From the very beginning, I felt like a survivor, not a victim," says Meili, 45, a slender, elegantly dressed woman with large gray-green eyes and short frosted hair.

She pushed herself through an accelerated rehabilitation and returned to Salomon despite not feeling 100% mentally or physically. She became vice president, a position she had coveted.

Meili even gathered the strength to testify at two criminal trials of the five teenagers accused of assaulting her. (Their convictions were later vacated when a convicted murderer claimed he was the sole attacker and DNA evidence put him at the scene.)

Although Meili had returned to her earlier life, it wasn't the same. She gradually felt a greater draw toward helping people like herself who faced disabilities and trauma. So she left the business world to take on this new mission. Now she's a motivational speaker and volunteer who talks about her healing to medical and mental health groups, patients and others recovering from traumatic changes.

Amazing as her recovery might appear, it makes perfect sense because Meili's personality and actions are a recipe for overcoming trauma, according to new research that shows what works best for anyone facing difficult challenges.

Among the key ingredients that create resilience:

A "can-do" optimism and goal setting. Raised with two older brothers, Meili was a scrappy kid. "I've been competitive and a fighter all my life," she says. Her efforts paid off, which built optimism. People who think they can get somewhere set goals and try harder, says psychologist George Bonanno of Columbia University.

There's also evidence that optimism helps ward off depression, which can sink people after crises, says psychologist Barbara Fredrickson of the University of Michigan. Meili set daily goals and drove herself relentlessly. Even small changes reinforce the "can-do" sense and keep one pushing forward, says psychologist Karen Reivich, co-author of The Resilience Factor.

A "present" emphasis. "I didn't wallow in 'what ifs' and 'if onlys'" Meili says. She knew she was in the fight of her life. "I felt I couldn't afford to dissolve in rage about the past or ruminate about the future." Depression and anxiety slow recovery, Reivich says, because they drain energy needed for healing. So it's best to stay in the present and make the most of it.

Bravery. Not the shoot-'em-up kind, but facing the hardest thing head-on. For Meili, it was her obvious, humiliating mental gaps. Intellectual ability "was the trait my family valued most" and her stock in trade. "I had to face this dragon," she says. She fought the beast every day with every memory and cognitive exercise at hand.

This kind of bravery increases the chances of recovering from traumas such as rape and assaults, according to a new study by Seligman and University of Michigan psychologist Christopher Peterson.

Willingness to accept help. Meili took pride in always being the strong one but quickly saw that she couldn't make it without throngs of helpers. She held on to all the outstretched hands, feeling gratitude. It's a myth that resilient people display a solitary toughness, says psychologist Salvatore Maddi of the University of California-Irvine. The best copers readily reach out for support when they need it, he says.

Spirituality and life-changing growth. Spirituality aids people in overcoming challenges, several studies show. And successful copers often develop a new mission, Reivich says. "They're glad they're still here but ask themselves, 'What am I doing with this blessing that I'm still here?'"

The best copers actually thrive under traumas that look daunting, says Maddi, whose pioneering research on what he called "the hardy personality" was ahead of its time in the 1980s. "Hardy people see challenge as a normal way of life and grow with it," Maddi says.

Trisha Meili fits the profile to a T. "I like myself better than I used to," she says. "I'm still a whole person, and in some ways a lot stronger than I was before."

Myths abound about resilience. One is that a positive attitude is merely denial, which prevents people from facing up to what has happened. Some thought she was in denial, Meili writes in her 2003 book, I Am the Central Park Jogger: A Story of Hope and Possibility. But she didn't feel in denial. She just wanted to move on ‹ as rapidly as possible.

People in denial hide under their covers: They get drunk, they avoid facing facts, Maddi says. Meili's positive spin didn't lead to distracting herself; she confronted problems and focused on solutions.

Of course, the young banker's positive attitude before the attack fostered recovery. But because genes influence disposition, not everyone is born with such a rosy outlook.

"To say something is partly heritable doesn't mean it's not changeable," Reivich says. Research shows people can learn ways to become resilient, she adds. They can practice techniques that help them stay in the present, keep things in perspective and work on the problems at hand.

Meili's is a story of mega-recovery. But her healing signposts can guide others facing less horrific, everyday challenges that still try the soul and body, Reivich says.

Meili hopes so. She says it heartens her to realize that she can make a difference in the lives of others, "just as others had made a difference in my recovery. . . . It doesn't matter what I could have been. What matters is who I am right now."

Psychologists have always been interested in how people survive trauma, especially massive traumatic events such as the events in World War II, the death camps set up by the Nazis, and the U.S. dropping the atomic bomb on Hiroshima and Nagasaki, and, more recently, terrorist bombings in cities throughout the world. We define a *survivor* as someone who has been exposed to the possibility of dying and/or who has witnessed the death of others, but remained alive and who makes some attempt to restore normalcy to his or her life. If there is no attempt made by the person to try to recover psychologically and get on with life, even if it cannot be as before, such as in Trisha Meili's account, then we say that person remains a *victim*.

Using these definitions, we see that a person can be both a victim and a survivor. The victim may not have control over what happened to him or her, but the survivor does have some control over what happens next. Any experience of crisis can connect the person with prior crisis, victimization, or survival. Sometimes the connections can be made from one crisis to another by similar experiences while, in other cases, the meanings from the crisis are constructed by that person or others. For example, many survivors of the holocaust during World War II have found recovery in combating other destructive and evil forces that remain in the world. Trisha Meili found psychological recovery in becoming a motivational speaker, using what she learned about resilience to help others who have experienced similar tragic events.

In some cases, collective survival missions can turn destructive and use the survivor's vengeful feelings to wage mass violence and war against others. For example, the current Jihad against the Western world by some Middle Eastern Muslims has become bound together with feelings of betrayal and injustice against those who are not of the same religious practices. Similar feelings may also be expressed by individuals such as seen in many serial killers who have experienced horrendous child abuse which they then turn into suspicion and hatred against others. Sometimes it is expressed against the abusers themselves, such as some patricide cases where children kill abusive parents, and sometimes it is expressed more diffusely, as in the case of the Unibomber who killed for alleged ideological beliefs; the DC sniper, John Allan Mohammed, who, together with his young companion, killed random people from his car; or even the young Palestinian suicide bombers who kill themselves as well as thousands of innocent people whom they have learned to hate.

Psychologist and author, Phyllis Chesler writes of the dangers of appeasement in her new book, published in 2006 and entitled *The Price of Appeasement*. Chesler compares the Palestinian intifada from 2000 to 2006 against Israel and the Jews to Hitler's genocidal intent in the period before 1940 when his terrorist acts spread to engulf most of the entire world. Chesler believes that the appeasement of any types of murderers especially those in totalitarian regimes such as found in the

Middle East Islamic countries, their terrorism will spread globally. She compares individual terrorism with those in organized groups noting that it is difficult for current and potential victims to assign blame directly to the terrorists, much like happens with abused children, battered women, and kidnapping victims who invariably blame themselves and try harder to appease their captors, hoping that this time they will stop their offending behavior. Chesler suggests that the solution is for the targeted victims to organize their response and fight back, beginning with exposing the behavior, labeling it as terrorism and connecting all such acts together so the destructive pattern is unmistakable.

Many people who work in the criminal justice system have difficulty when psychologists try to understand the mental state of those who commit these horrendous acts, especially when innocent people are killed. Often they fear that a mental health defense will be successful and, therefore, the crimes will go unpunished. This can happen, of course, especially if the perpetrators are so mentally ill they do not understand that what they have done is against the law and has negative consequences. That is the purpose of the insanity defense—not to allow people to escape punishment but, rather, to help restore someone's competency or sanity. Punishment is useless in cases where people are so mentally ill that they can't understand why they are being punished. We still may have to protect society by placing them in a forensic hospital until they are no longer dangerous. Usually this means a much longer time being held in a locked ward in a state forensic hospital than these people would have spent in prison if they had been convicted. People in these hospitals have fewer rights or privileges than if they were in prison. However, in most of the cases where people are using violence against others after having been victimized themselves, individually or in a group, they do not meet the insanity statutes but, rather, may just need to be better understood, both to help them heal in a more socially responsible way and to protect society from any further vengeful violence.

It is important to remember that people can continue to experience the crisis either in reality, in virtual reality, or through the reexperiencing of the event(s) in their own mind. It is common to reexperience crisis events that are traumatic if people are then exposed to similar stimuli, if there is exposure to closely related stimuli, if the trauma is stimulated by memory, or if there are internal stimuli that set off the trauma memories. If these reexperiences last up to one month, this is called an *Acute Stress Disorder (ASD)*, and, if it is longer, then it is called a *Post Traumatic Stress Disorder (PTSD)*. PTSD has been described in an earlier chapter on anxiety disorders because it is classified in that way by the diagnostic systems. See Chapter 7 for the criteria used to make a diagnosis. PTSD is the most common psychological reaction following a trauma or crisis event, and, therefore, it will be further described here.

CRISIS

The definition of a *crisis* is the perception or experience of an event or situation as intolerable and something that exceeds the person's current resources and coping mechanisms. Crisis has the potential to cause severe cognitive, affective, and behavioral malfunctioning if there is no relief. Crisis also has the potential to cause disorganization, disruption, upset, fear, shock, and immobilization among other feelings and thoughts. Crisis brings with it both the presence of danger and the possibility of the opportunity for change. People may cope with their pain independently and survive, but block any potential growth, or break down until the crisis is resolved. There may be complicated symptomology that occurs together with normally expected crisis reactions, especially if this is not the first crisis experienced by the person. It is important to know as much as possible about the person, as well as about the crisis situation, in order to maximize help during the crisis, especially if there are idiosyncratic reactions to the situation. However, it is possible to intervene in crisis situations, even without knowing much about the individual involved, especially in seriously traumatic situations. Most crisis periods offer the opportunity for people to change and grow in ways that may have been thought about previously, but, for whatever reasons, seemed too difficult for the individual at the previous time.

Types of Crises

Typical crises may be expected in a person's life while other crises are unexpected and sometimes traumatic.

Developmental crises are normal during the life cycle of an individual. These may include when a child is born or taken into a family, when a death occurs, when someone gets married, leaves home, or graduates from school. Adjustment reactions of adolescence and other normal developmental crisis periods are diagnoses that reflect the inability to resolve these normal, developmental, life-cycle types of crises. They usually, but not always, have mild symptoms, but they may last longer than expected and have an impact on various functions.

Situational crises are uncommon and even extraordinary events. They tend to be random, sudden, shocking, intense, and even catastrophic at times. The most difficult to deal with are situational crises that are brought about by other people in our lives who then have the power to change our lives in unanticipated ways, for example, if a husband comes home and announces that he wants a divorce when there had not been any previous discussion of marital problems.

Existential crises occur when something either inside in the mind or in the external reality of people's lives causes them to rethink all their values and ideals. It may be a crisis of faith, of moral values, or just a rethinking of all that a person believes in. For example, it may be as

BOX 10.2

Autonomic Nervous System Crisis Pathway

ANS is activated → neuroendocrine system secretes more or less of the neurotransmitters → causing damage to the brain structure(s), particularly the hippocampal area → impacting on memory encoding and consolidation → and stimuli associated with past events are activated → developing new sights, sounds, smells, and visual images that will reactivate this pathway and restimulate the ANS without the original stimulus of stress, crisis or trauma being present.

dramatic as a POW's being tortured or as prosaic as a woman's falling in love with a married man. More often than not, it occurs alone rather than with groups of others experiencing the same crisis.

Environmental crises occur when something in the environment occurs that is so traumatic that it produces a major psychological reaction. Trauma and violence are in this category, as is other family maltreatment such as child, elder, and intimate partner abuse. They may be repeated traumas that finally rise to the level of crisis or smaller abusive situations that finally reach a threshold where some protective action must be taken.

Transcrisis states include various unresolved crises that limit a person's functioning to a minimal level. This is different from a crisis that was resolved at the time it occurred, but the psychological impact recurs when a new crisis is similar to, or reminds one of, the earlier crisis. Someone who has not resolved one or more crises may be said to be in a transcrisis state.

PHYSIOLOGICAL RESPONSE TO CRISIS AND TRAUMA

Crises, especially those that involve some type of traumatic event, often produce a physiological response similar to what stress does to the mind and body. Generally this physiological response is triggered by the *autonomic nervous system (ANS)* that was described in Chapter 4 when the brain and nervous system, which controls the physiological responses to stress, crises, and trauma, were discussed. The crisis pathway can be found in Box 10.2.

What activates in the neuroendocrine system?

The hippocampal area, which is activated in the neuroendocrine response to stress, crisis, and trauma, included brain structures that manufacture some of the neurotransmitters, as well as other areas of the body that manufacture and store other neuromodulators and hormones. Hormones are part of the body's endocrine system that are manufactured and stored, only to be released when they are needed. They usually get to the brain and nervous system through the blood system. One neurotransmitter that is particularly important in this ANS stress,

Table 10.1. Autonomic Nervous System Physiological Response

- Increases heart rate
- Increases blood pressure
- Increases triglycerides
- Increases cholesterol
- Decreases blood flow to the skin
- Decreases blood flow to gastrointestinal area
- Decreases blood flow to renal area
- Activates the neuroendocrine system (see Box 10.2)

crisis, and trauma pathway is called *cortisol*. Researchers are studying the effects of cortisol on the body's resilience to stress because it appears that too much or too little can make a big difference in how someone reacts to the crisis. In Chapter 4 we discussed the body's ability to upregulate or downregulate, meaning to manufacture more or less of a chemical substance when its sensors indicate too little or too much is available. In this case, too little cortisol may be sensed, causing the body to release too much, in turn, causing part of the ANS's crisis pathway responses. It is important to realize that these ANS responses occur automatically, without someone's thought patterns influencing them. See Table 10.1 for a list of physiological responses to stress.

Fight or Flight Response to Danger

When danger is perceived and a person becomes afraid, the ANS and its physiological responses are activated. High levels of arousal occur when the neuroendocrine system's chemicals are flooding the various parts of the brain and rest of the body, causing them to deal with whatever is frightening the person. There is usually observable anxiety, hypervigilance, startle reaction, intense preoccupation with what is occurring and less ability to notice or concentrate on anything else, physiological disruption, and discomfort within the body. The goal is self-protection which is usually accomplished by fighting the dangerous enemy or getting away (flight). Psychologists who specialize in crisis and trauma have learned how to measure the fight responses by assessing for specific patterns of anxiety that are commonly observed in victims and survivors. It is important to remember that the purpose of these reactions is self-protective, not to hurt someone else. For example, battered women who kill their abuser often do so in response to terrifying fear that causes this self-protective response. Today these women are usually permitted to obtain a psychologist to evaluate them, and, if the appropriate signs and symptoms are present, they may be able to use the fact that they have developed what is called Battered Woman Syndrome as part of the evidence that they acted in what they believed was self defense. We discuss this further later in this chapter.

The most natural response to facing a terrifying threat of danger is to run away—the flight part of this response. However, what happens if the person is unable to run away, like in a crisis situation? If physical flight is not possible, there is always mental flight. Mentally removing oneself from a dangerous situation is also done automatically, without conscious thought. Psychologists name the different mental processes that can occur. They are called denial, minimization, avoidance, depression, repression, and dissociation. Some of these processes are the same ones that occur in other mental illnesses. However, they also can be used by non-mentally ill people in situations that require them. For example, most of us have learned to avoid doing something that is distasteful to us. In this case, avoidance is purposeful and intentionally used after some thought or cognitive process. Sometimes, however, it is not necessary to think about avoiding something that is dangerous. Think about the reflex responses that occur when something hot is touched, like on the stove, and the person's hand immediately pulls away to avoid getting burned. These ANS mediated flight responses are activated without cognitive thought, and like the reflex response, they occur as self-protection.

Let us take a look at some of these mental flight responses since they will be important to recognize when working with someone in crisis.

Denial occurs when people are aware of what has happened or is still happening, but they are afraid that they cannot accept it and so deny that it has happened to them or someone else. The difference between denial and a lie is that denial is unconscious while a lie is purposeful. Both may be used for self preservation, but they are different processes.

Minimization occurs when people are aware that there is danger out there, but minimize it so that their fear is lowered, and they are not paralyzed into inaction. Sometimes minimization is accompanied with some bravado, like "I can handle that dangerous situation without any help."

Avoidance can be conscious or unconscious. It occurs when someone no longer gets pleasure out of doing what he or she used to like to do and, therefore, no longer does it. For example, if a person witnessed a car accident at a particular corner while going home that person might stay away from the site and take a different route without even realizing that she or he was avoiding the other route home. Rape victims often avoid doing something that might remind them of the trauma they experienced. A "trauma trigger" is something that takes on the same emotional fears as what caused the trauma originally, and is responsible for re-experiencing the trauma response. An aroma that is similar to the one that a rapist was wearing at the time of the assault might become a trauma trigger for that victim. Should someone else be wearing the same scent, it might cause the woman to begin acting as if she were being raped again.

Conscious avoidance is different from avoidance behaviors that the person is unaware of. Conscious avoidance often occurs when a battered woman tries to please her partner so that he does not abuse her at that time. This can get complicated, however, when the battered woman recognizes that the abuse will occur anyway, and tries to find a safe time or place to experience the acute battering incident. Sometimes the woman may precipitate an explosion by the batterer so others are around and can protect her when the batterer starts harming her.

Dissociation is another psychological process that occurs when people have experienced such horrifying trauma that they separate the mind from the body so as not to feel the physical and emotional pain. It is a trance-like process in that people may seem as if they know what is happening on one level of consciousness, but, on another level, the cognitive mind simply shuts down. Child abuse victims often go into a dissociative state during the abuse by making their mind think about something else so they do not pay attention to the abuse they are receiving. Many sexual abuse survivors relate staring at a crack in the ceiling or a picture on the wall in order to distract themselves from what is happening to their bodies.

Repression is another unconscious psychological process whereby a negative experience is shut out of the conscious mind so the pain associated with it is not experienced. Unacceptable memories are then repressed in the unconscious mind. *Psychoanalysis* was developed as one way to make these memories conscious and available to the patients who often were not aware of them.

Today we have many different types of crisis intervention and therapy that try to help people cope with the aftermath of crisis and trauma. There has been a debate more recently about the nature of repressed memories and whether what is uncovered in therapy is an actual memory or something the therapist had implanted in the client's mind. Some forms of treatment that encourage reliving the memories and changing what really happened in one's mind, like beating up abusers or shrinking them in size in one's mind, have been implicated in helping clients develop false memories of abuse. However, there is no scientific evidence that it is possible to implant a false trauma memory. Most people do not repress all of a traumatic childhood, nor do they accept someone else's intentional or unintentional attempts to implant false memories about what happened to them. Rather, it appears that they may not have the ability to reexperience painful emotions all of the time and, so, sometimes they repress the memories while other times those memories come to the surface.

Basic Crisis Theory for Interventions

It is important to differentiate between a crisis reaction, an Acute Stress Disorder, and Post Traumatic Stress Disorder, which can be acute, chronic, or complex. In addition, the multiple axis system of the DSM allows for diagnosis of other disorders simultaneously, although

Table 10.2. Steps to Resolving a Crisis

Five important steps:

1. Identify grief responses to loss, which can be tangible or intangible such as loss of quality of life, different internal feelings, or self-image.
2. Assess impediments, if any, for the person to attain life goals.
3. Recognize and correct temporary distortions produced by crisis such as those in the cognitive, affective, and behavioral domains.
4. Help the client reorganize and resolve the crisis.
5. Assess for residual effects even after the crisis is resolved.

Five normal stages of grief after a crisis are:

1. There is a preoccupation with the lost person or goal.
2. There is identification with the lost person or goal and an attempt to fix or even get out of the situation.
3. There are feelings and expressions of guilt and hostility such as anger at the system or others involved in whatever set off the crisis.
4. There is usually some disorganization in daily routine. This might be real such as being put in jail or some other change in lifestyle.
5. There may be evidence of somatic complaints that often accompany crisis.

it is usually a good idea to wait until the crisis passes before making a diagnosis. When assessing the psychological impact of a crisis, it is important to determine if it is an acute or chronic state of crisis, as well as the person's current level of functioning. This would include the emotional or affective severity, the cognitive status, and the behavioral function such as approach-avoidance conflicts and paralysis if they exist. Table 10.2 suggests steps that are usually taken when using crisis theory with grief responses.

There are different psychological theories that may be useful to assist a person in resolving a crisis situation. See Box 10.3 for a description of them.

THE HAZARDS OF HELPING: EMOTIONAL TRAUMA AND TREATMENT INTERVENTIONS FOR FIRST RESPONDERS

First Responders, including police, firefighters, paramedics, and dispatchers, are themselves especially vulnerable to stress, trauma and the resulting crisis response. Unlike most other professions, First Responders constantly face the possibility of gunfire, conflagrations that result in collapsing buildings or explosions, life or death decisions in emergency medical treatment that could, in some instances, cause them to contract disease, terrorist attacks, or the responsibility to give

---

BOX 10.3

Crisis Theories for Intervention

Psychoanalytic theory understands disequilibrium produced in crisis through the access to unconscious thoughts and past emotions with emphasis on early childhood.

Psychoadaptional theory suggests understanding and changing maladaptive behaviors by learning to change negative thoughts through adaptive and positive coping.

Systems theory states that all elements are interrelated in the ecological system and if you change one part then you must expect change in another part, which will permit the resolution of the crisis.

Interpersonal theory suggests resolution of the crisis by enhancing self-esteem, openness, trust, sharing, safety, unconditional positive regard, and empathy.

Chaos theory states that chaos is really predictable scientifically, or even if not, it gives the opportunity for change and growth if the person's anxiety can be calmed down. Francine Shapiro, founder of EMDR (Eye Move Desensitization and Reprocessing), suggests that non-linear, spontaneous, random, unfolding, non-cause and effect behaviors can organize into new patterns.

Feminist theory suggests that there is a build up of feelings and cognitions that are associated with oppression from discrimination that impact on crisis resolution. Reempowerment or the regaining of personal power and belief in one's own self-efficacy are associated with recovery.

Trauma theory suggests that responses to trauma are usually normal behaviors needed to respond to an abnormal situation. Regaining feelings of self-efficacy and power are associated with recovery.

Equilibrium theory suggests that restoring equilibrium early in the crisis is the best way to recover from crisis.

Cognitive theory suggests changing beliefs about facts and situations that surround the crisis, especially self-talk, will resolve crisis states. Re-wiring and developing new positive feedback loops will help once there is stabilization.

Psychosocial Transition theory assesses internal and external facts of crisis and then develops a plan to determine what a person needs to effectively resolve the crisis such as better internal coping, more support systems, access to more environmental resources, etc which is best after stabilization.

Survivor theory suggests that victims need to take back their power to heal from crisis. It is a combination of feminist and trauma theories.

---

directions over the phone on saving a drowning child's life. *Critical incidents* like these can cause psychological crises and potentially PTSD. It is important for crisis workers to be aware of the possibility that they may be struggling with the emotional impact of their work.

A *Critical Incident* is any event that has the emotional power to overwhelm First Responders' usual ability to cope and that may impede the functioning of their coping skills either immediately or in the future. Critical incidents include exposure to homicides, rapes, robberies, assaults, serious accidents, acts of terrorism, and natural disasters. Often the normal coping mechanisms fail individuals exposed to critical incidents. These incidents are usually quite specific and time-limited; they cause acute stress and may involve loss or threat to personal goals or well-being. Experiencing a critical incident could be a turning point in someone's life. It is experienced by direct or primary victims, but can also be experienced as trauma by witnesses to these painful incidents, which can produce secondary victims.

Table 10.3. Characteristics of Effective Crisis Workers

1. Successful resolution of their own life experiences.
2. Professional skills such as attentiveness, listening skills, congruence, ability to be supportive, think analytically, and problem solving skills such as assessment and ability to make appropriate referrals.
3. Stability and poise.
4. Creativity and flexibility.
5. Energy.
6. Quick mental resources.
7. Multicultural competencies such as knowing:
   a. Assumption of what is normal behavior varies from culture to culture.
   b. The individual is not the most important part of all societies.
   c. Identities of helpers need to include qualities other than academic qualities.
   d. Abstract constructs are not always the same in all cultures.
   e. Independence is not the most valued goal in all cultures.
   f. Informal therapy may be just as important or even more so that formal therapy.
   g. Scientific cause and effect is not the explanation that all parts of the world believe in, especially in places that believe in supernatural and metaphysical events.
   h. The system and not necessarily the individual must change if there is a bad fit.
   i. The client's past history does matter, even during a crisis.
   j. It is important to know what you do and do not know about someone else's culture.

Table 10.4. Six Steps in Crisis Theory

1. Define the problem
2. Secure the person's safety
3. Provide support
4. Examine alternatives
5. Make plans for the future
6. Obtain commitment

There are a number of characteristics that are considered to be important for an effective crisis worker to have. They are suggested in Table 10.3.

Finally, Table 10.4 lists the major steps to be followed in resolving a crisis situation.

All First Responders who are involved in such situations remain vulnerable. The majority of First Responders who encounter a critical incident do not develop full blown PTSD with the attendant symptoms of flashbacks or nightmares. More typically, they may experience emotional numbing, withdrawal from social and family involvement, denial of feelings and increased use of alcohol or drugs. To avert these problems, clinicians and researchers have developed a number of interventions designed to prevent or mitigate the crisis response and enable the First Responders to cope effectively with the trauma.

CRITICAL INCIDENT STRESS MANAGEMENT (CISM)

Perhaps the best known program used following a crisis is the Critical Incident Stress Management (CISM) model used by law enforcement and other First Responders after an incident has occurred. CISM is an integrated, multi-component, crisis intervention model that deals with the pre-crisis, acute crisis, and post crisis phases. It is well thought out both in theory and practice, although its success is difficult to measure given the varied situations in which it is practiced. The goal of CISM is to minimize *acute* psychological distress and prevent or mediate the intensity of post trauma sequelae. The theory evolved from the work of Kardiner and Spiegel who studied military crises and intervention with military personnel, Lindeman's studies on transition through the crisis of grief, Erikson's work on normal developmental issues, and Caplan's crisis work in emotionally hazardous situations.

A comprehensive stress management program will involve the recruitment of a CISM team that is composed of carefully selected personnel, from inside as well as outside the organization, who themselves are emotionally stable and capable of dealing with the stress situations that they will face. This team will be involved in pre-crisis, acute crisis and post crisis phases of the program.

Pre-Crisis Phase

The pre-crisis phase of the program focuses on anticipatory planning and clear information about each person's job expectations and disaster protocols. Personnel need to be oriented to the potential stressors they will face in any situation in order to establish clear expectations and to develop a mindset that will help to eliminate confusion and disorganization that would impair performance. Additionally, personnel should be introduced to information about stress, its effects on the body and emotions, and typical stress reactions as well as skills and community resources in managing stress.

Acute Crisis Phase

The CISM team can provide an array of support services during the actual trauma or disaster that are basic actions that provide an emotional safety net for personnel, enabling them to deal with their stressors more effectively. Structuring of work tasks that can be rotated to minimize fatigue; provision of food, water and clean clothes; a clear chain of command, and frequent updates on the status of the situation;

rest periods; and removal of First Responders from the situation when they manifest signs of decompensation are all helpful steps to be taken in the midst of the traumatic event.

Post Crisis Phase

Demobilizations are very brief mini informational sessions given to small groups of First Responders who are removed from the immediate disaster site, given some basic support and information about their potential for a stress reaction, provided basic food, water and rest, and sent away from the disaster for at least twelve hours. This intervention is designed to provide basic information about potential stress reactions in order to "tide them over" until a full *Debriefing* can be held several days later. Those identified during this intervention as needing additional help may be given individual attention.

Defusings involve the CISM team's providing a brief forum to a group of First Responders to discuss informally the traumatic event they have experienced together relatively soon after it has occurred. It represents a prelude to a full debriefing and, in some instances, may eliminate the need for a more extensive session. Here also, the team provides information about expected stress reactions and ways to cope with them effectively.

Critical Incident Stress Debriefing is a very specific intervention that is employed after a traumatic event. It is designed not only to minimize the acute stress but also to be a prophylaxis against future stress reactions. In a major disaster, the debriefing will follow a demobilization by a couple of weeks. See Table 10.5 for the core elements of this model.

A *CISD* intervention usually includes debriefing of individuals or in groups as a cornerstone. The typical process can be found in Table 10.6.

Group Debriefing was developed to help crisis workers in lowering their own reactions to stress. The goals are similar to other forms of crisis intervention to prevent maladaptive responses to critical acts and to stabilize, restore feelings of mastery, and develop support networks. It is

Table 10.5. Core Elements of Critical Incident Stress Management (CISM)

1. Pre crisis preparation (individuals and organizations).
2. Large scale mobilization and demobilization procedures for large scale disasters.
3. Individual acute crisis counseling available.
4. Small group discussions for the acute phase that are brief are the primary means of dissemination of information and discussion of feelings.
5. Small group discussions that are longer including Critical Incident Stress Debriefing (CISD) which is a trademark of this intervention especially with crisis workers to prevent further emotional harm to them.
6. Family crisis intervention techniques when entire families are involved.
7. Follow up procedures and referral for long term therapy where needed.

Table 10.6. The Typical CISD Process Model

1. Intervening immediately
2. Listening to the facts of the event
3. Encouraging ventilation of feelings
4. Reflection of victims' feelings
5. Consolation and comfort to victims
6. Gaining a perspective on the situation
7. Taking direct, reality-based actions
8. Facilitating social support

Table 10.7. Mitchell's CISD Model for Groups

1. Facts of critical incident are clearly established as known
2. First the thoughts of the group members are discussed
3. Then discuss emotions of the group members
4. Discuss any PTSD symptoms that group members have experienced
5. Strategies to cope with additional stress are discussed
6. Prepare crisis workers to return to their usual life with psychological closure

based on the goals of immediacy, proximity, and expectancy. There are two main models—one developed by Mitchell and modified by Dyregov, and one developed by Raphael.

Mitchell's model integrates emotional and cognitive experiences of crisis in the debriefing. The model requires group process in the debriefing, usually two to seven days post crisis, and the group session is planned to last two to three hours. However, there could be defusing on the same day of the incident. The Mitchell model can be found in Table 10.7.

Dyregov added some process variables to Mitchell's model, focusing on the decision-making process of participants. It also adds discussion of the stage of sensory impressions of the incident that were experienced and emphasizes the normalization of the reactions and responses.

The *Raphael Model* focuses on emotional experiences of participants and doesn't have a formal cognitive piece as does the Mitchell model. It discusses preparedness prior to the event that might influence perceptions during it. The individual's own role and experience during the event is usually processed right after the incident so that positive and negative experiences can be processed. The focus is on the interpersonal relationships during the event, including possible identification with the victims, impact on friendships, impact on family relationships, etc. Like the other models, the final goal is the transition back to normal life. The general features of the group include development of various group processes such as group cohesion, catharsis, imitative behavior, sharing information, and addressing existential issues. The group is expected to share emotional impact by ventilating and *carthartic abre-action,* which is the analytic term for emotional release. This method emphasizes the building of caring attachments through supportive networks and adaptive coping responses which are expected to develop in the cognitive and behavioral domains.

Critics of the CISM Models

There have been criticisms of the CISM models from mental health experts who are trying to develop a way to measure treatment efficacy. For example, on September 6, 2002. *The Washington Post* headlined an article that cited two studies that questioned whether debriefings and counseling after a trauma are good or if they might even be harmful, using the experiences after September 11 and a Dutch study across multiple traumas. Obviously, it is difficult to study the efficacy of this intervention given the large numbers of people whom it reaches and the minimal information obtained about them prior to the trauma and subsequent crisis intervention. Although many First Responders recommend using CISM after a trauma, some people may only need information and a place to vent feelings for a short period of time, while others will need much more care, especially if they do develop a PTSD afterwards. At present we do not have a way to screen those who are at high risk for PTSD, and so we follow the suggested approach from the mental health prevention field, and give everyone exposed to the trauma the same intervention.

It is also important not to confuse CISM with the evidence-based treatment movement in mental health since it does not lend itself easily to such analysis. For example, CISM is often performed by First Responders in crisis situations where it is almost impossible to assess all the variables impinging on any crisis worker at that time. The training of these emergency and relief workers is variable, so that the actual models as were described above may not be achieved from site to site. Psychologist Elizabeth Carll emphasized the political nature of some disasters, such as an international airline crash (TWA 800) and September 11 as compared to local homicides, home invasions or fires, and suggested there might be major differences in how politics affect the disaster relief offered.

It is important to remember that crisis intervention strategies, including CISM, are not the same as psychotherapy, even though some of the techniques might be similar. Rather, crisis strategies are designed to deal with the emotional impact of the traumatic event and are not considered long-term treatment. Some of the earlier discussion about regulating hormones such as Cortisol Releasing Factor that trigger the ANS into immediate action when danger is experienced could possibly

BOX 10.4

Comparison of Crisis Intervention & Psychotherapy

Crisis Intervention	*Psychotherapy*
Principles	
Diagnosis is rapid	Diagnosis is complete
Treatment focuses on immediate Trauma & impact on person	Treatment focuses on underlying causes— impact on entire person
Plan is problem-specific & symptoms	Plan is personalized with long term goals
Methods are brief, short-term, crisis goals	Systematic short & long term goals
Evaluation is of client pre-crisis	Evaluation is total functioning of client
Objectives	
Define problems	Prevent problems
Ensure client safety	Change ecological system
Provide support	Systematic support
Examine alternatives	Facilitate growth
Develop a plan	Reeducate
Obtain commitment	Express and clarify emotions
	Resolve conflict
	Accept reality
	Maximize resources
Assess Client Functioning	
Intake data—brief	Intake data when stable & in depth
Safety—first concern	Safety issues not usually primary
Time—urgency	Time not so urgent & slower planning
Reality test—simple	Assumes reality unless reason not to
Referrals—pick up immediately	Referrals assumed to be longer time
Consultation—on call	Consultation—assume crisis not needed
Drug use—assess self-report & visual	Drug use—treatment data & random testing

prevent PTSD. Crisis intervention techniques can prevent more serious psychological problems from developing if done within a short time after the crisis has occurred. See Box 10.4 for a comparison of crisis intervention and psychotherapy.

CHRONIC vs. ACUTE STRESS

While the dramatic and overwhelming trauma and disasters described above give rise to acute stress that may be best addressed with CISM, most First Responders will not face this type of situation in their careers. Rather, they will face day to day stressors that build up insidiously over time and ultimately erode their coping ability and numb their sensitivity to their own as well as others' feelings. For instance, police officers make routine traffic stops everyday. While most are routine, officers must constantly be on guard for violence and must decide how to approach each situation. Police department standards may demand that the officer be very courteous and friendly to avoid citizen complaints, but expect constant vigilance to avoid dropping one's guard. The incompatibility of these approaches can result in chronic stress.

Law enforcement personnel are constantly faced with assessing many other highly complex scenarios requiring them to make snap decisions. They must also follow departmental standard operating procedures or face disciplinary action. The result of these potential conflicts is chronic stress. Other more mundane stressful events including being passed over for a promotion, responding to the death of a child, suspension, long hours, and extended time away from family contribute to the chronic stress endured by many First Responders. The emotional fallout that comes from confronting these stressors results in police having one of the highest suicide rates, a high divorce rate, serious substance abuse problems, and a high incidence of domestic violence.

SUGGESTED READINGS

Barbanel, L. & Sternberg, R. J. (2006). *Psychological interventions in times of crisis*. New York: Springer.

Carll, E. K. (2004). Critical Incident Stress Intervention following disaster: Helpful or Iatrogenic. *The Independent Practitioner: Bulletin of the Psychologists in Independent Practice of the American Psychological Association, 24(1)*, 11–14.

Campfield, K. M. & Hills, A. M. (2001). Effect of timing of Critical Incident Stress Debriefing (CISD) on Posttraumatic symptoms. *Journal of Traumatic Stress, 14(2)*, 327–340.

Figley, C. R. (Ed.). (1995). *Compassion fatigue: Coping with secondary PTSD in those who treat the traumatized*. New York: Brunner/Mazel.

Greene, P., Kane, D., Christ, G., Lynch, S., & Corrigan, M. (2006). *FDNY Crisis Counseling: Innovative responses to 911 firefighters, families, & communities*. New York: Wiley.

James, R. K. & Gilliland, B. E. (2001). *Crisis intervention strategies: Fourth Edition*. Stamford, CT: Brooks/Cole/Wadsworth/Thomson Learning Academic Resource Center.

La Grecca, A. M., Sevin, S. W., & Sevin, E. L. (2005). *After the storm: A guide to help children cope with the psychological effects of a hurricane*. Coral Gables, FL: 7-Dippity, Inc.

Meichenbaum, D. (1994). *A clinical handbook/Practical therapist manual for assessing and treating adults with Post-Traumatic Stress Disorder (PTSD)*. Waterloo, Ontario, CN: Institute Press.

Van Hasselt, V. B., Baker, M. T., Dalfonzo, V. A., Romano, S. J., Schlessinger, K. M., Zucker, M., Dragone, R., & Perera, A. L. (2005). Crisis (hostage) negotiation Training: A preliminary evaluation of program efficacy. *Criminal Justice & Behavior*.

CHAPTER 11

Therapeutic Justice

Therapeutic Justice, Restorative Justice, and *Problem-Solving Courts* are names given by the criminal justice system to diversion programs that attempt to help people with serious mental illnesses get therapeutic intervention rather than languish in jails and prisons. As we have stated earlier, the statistics in the United States as well as the rest of the world indicate that more and more defendants in criminal proceedings enter the criminal justice system with previously diagnosed mental illnesses, ranging from schizophrenia and mood disorders to substance abuse problems. In fact, recent data from the U.S. Department of Justice suggest that approximately one-half of all defendants have been diagnosed with a mental illness by the time they are arrested, and approximately 60% of all defendants have substance abuse problems that may have gotten them in trouble with the law. Approximately 6.4% have a serious mental illness, with women, who make up only approximately 11% of jail inmates, having twice as many such disorders. In addition, women who are arrested are more likely to enter jails with multiple other problems that stem from their child raising responsibilities and histories of domestic violence, sexual abuse, and other trauma experiences. One-third of women defendants have been found to suffer from Post Traumatic Stress Disorder (PTSD) at some point in their lives.

As a result, the criminal justice system has attempted jail diversion and intervention programs for people with serious mental illness and co-occurring substance abuse disorders, using models such as drug, domestic violence, and mental health specialty courts. In many cases, defendants are permitted to volunteer for such diversion programs directly from their court of first appearance. The data from a large, urban, Southern Florida magistrates' court are presented in Boxes 11.1a and 11.1b.

In many communities, the services for substance abusers and the mentally ill have been curtailed due to budgetary restraints, so many of the same people who might have found help in outpatient community mental health centers or inpatient state hospitals now find themselves

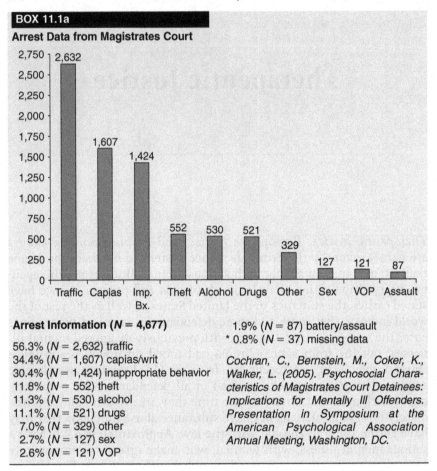

BOX 11.1a

Arrest Data from Magistrates Court

Arrest Information (N = 4,677)

56.3% (N = 2,632) traffic
34.4% (N = 1,607) capias/writ
30.4% (N = 1,424) inappropriate behavior
11.8% (N = 552) theft
11.3% (N = 530) alcohol
11.1% (N = 521) drugs
7.0% (N = 329) other
2.7% (N = 127) sex
2.6% (N = 121) VOP

1.9% (N = 87) battery/assault
* 0.8% (N = 37) missing data

Cochran, C., Bernstein, M., Coker, K., Walker, L. (2005). Psychosocial Characteristics of Magistrates Court Detainees: Implications for Mentally Ill Offenders. Presentation in Symposium at the American Psychological Association Annual Meeting, Washington, DC.

incarcerated for minor crimes such as stealing food, walking with an opened can of beer, loitering and trespassing, driving without proper identification or insurance, and other similar behavior. In some jurisdictions, those who are homeless may engage purposely in similar behavior so they can be arrested and placed in jail where they will get hot food, medicine, and a safe bed to sleep in. However, most agree that these people do not need to be in jail; rather, they need social service intervention to get access to proper food, medication, therapy, housing, and other services. The U.S. President's 2003 New Freedom Commission on Mental Health report strongly supports the use of diversion programs to meet the needs of these people.

In addition to pre and post booking diversion programs for the mentally ill, which are new, if those who were arrested were declared Incompetent-to-Proceed to Trial because their mental illness prevents them from cooperating with their attorney or understanding the justice system, then those persons are transferred from the Department of

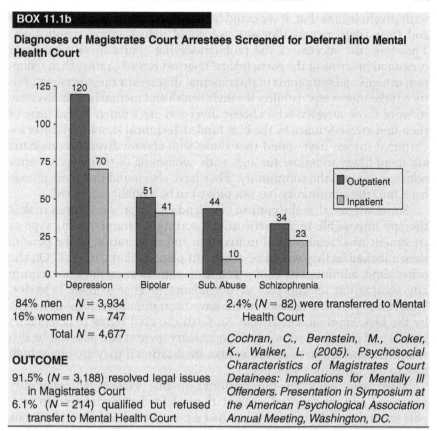

BOX 11.1b

Diagnoses of Magistrates Court Arrestees Screened for Deferral into Mental Health Court

84% men   N = 3,934
16% women N =   747

Total N = 4,677

OUTCOME

91.5% (N = 3,188) resolved legal issues in Magistrates Court

6.1% (N = 214) qualified but refused transfer to Mental Health Court

2.4% (N = 82) were transferred to Mental Health Court

Cochran, C., Bernstein, M., Coker, K., Walker, L. (2005). Psychosocial Characteristics of Magistrates Court Detainees: Implications for Mentally Ill Offenders. Presentation in Symposium at the American Psychological Association Annual Meeting, Washington, DC.

Corrections to the care of the Department of Social Services (or whoever is responsible for the care and treatment of the mentally ill in that community) and a program to restore their competency is begun. Often, seriously mentally ill people are unable to have their competency restored, and they may be released back into the community, supposedly with a plan for their own safety and others. If they are deemed dangerous to themselves or others, then they may be involuntarily committed to a hospital until such time as they are no longer suffering from the mental illness that had an impact on their criminal behavior. The process of involuntary civil commitment is discussed later in this chapter along with a discussion of new sex predator commitment laws that permit prison officials to recommend civil commitment of sexual predators to locked facilities for treatment after their prison terms are completed.

DOES REHABILITATION WORK?

While there are generally two sides of the argument, whether rehabilitation or treatment in jails and prisons work, most criminologists agree with psychologists that, if we could help people stay off alcohol and drugs and treat their mental illnesses, we could reduce crime significantly. Therefore, the success of the problem-solving courts mostly has been measured in terms of the participants' re-arrest records, rather than reduction in signs and symptoms of their mental illnesses or these persons' ability to take more responsibility for their health and mental health. Even so, most of those arrested who choose diversion are women at the time of their first arrest. Studies by the U.S. funded Technical Resource Center for Criminal Justice have found that those who choose diversion programs are more likely to follow through with counseling or therapy even after release back into the community. They have also found that their release back into the community has not proved to be a public safety risk.

Some suggest that the control of defendants in prison settings makes therapy impossible in an institutional setting. Certainly, if the type of treatment used requires full motivation and cooperation of the person, then a locked facility would be a difficult place to make it work. On the other hand, administration of psychotropic medication does not require any motivation on the part of defendants to change their behavior. During the past few decades, there have been important legal decisions by the U.S. Supreme Court that set forth the civil rights of defendants in jails and prisons, both to obtain necessary mental and physical health treatment and not to be forced to take medication if they are not at high risk to use dangerous violence.

Staff who work in the criminal justice system are generally untrained and unequipped to treat these defendants/prisoners. In fact, past mental health treatment has had a poor record in jails and prisons because it mostly dealt with improving prisoners' self-esteem, which is a difficult construct to measure, much less change. Today, new treatment programs have been designed that are focused on behavioral change and building self-efficacy in the prisoner—self efficacy being defined as the ability to do what is expected of the person and perform it properly and with self-confidence. These treatment programs have a far greater success record, but they are expensive to run and, therefore, rarely are enough of them found in the jails and prisons.

DRUG COURTS

The first of these therapeutic courts to be created was the drug court where those who are addicted to alcohol or other drugs can be sent for intervention rather than jail time. It became important to separate those who were selling illegal drugs from those who were using or abusing drugs when deferring into drug court. It has been recognized that some of the economic crimes that drug addicts committed were due to their addictions and, therefore, their recovery would help in preventing recidivism. The success of these courts relied upon their meeting minimum criteria such as frequent judicial status conferences, mandatory drug treatment, random drug screenings, negative sanctions for non-compliance, and positive rewards for achievements. Unfortunately, many of those addicted to alcohol and other drugs also have other mental health issues, necessitating dual diagnosis treatment centers rather than those just focused on substance abuse alone.

Most drug courts handle those defendants with misdemeanor, and sometimes felony, charges arising from use of illegal substances provided they were just using and not selling drugs. If they volunteer to be deferred into drug court, defendants are offered treatment rather than jail time for drug offenses. Usually those with alcohol and other drug habits are sent into local outpatient treatment programs with close supervision by the court. Case managers or probation workers who have been trained in alcohol and drug treatment are assigned to these courts; the judges usually volunteer for duty there, and, in some cases, there are psychologists and social workers who are available for further evaluation and referrals. Understanding that alcohol and drug treatment is difficult and often has many reversals before the individual is finally free of all substances, these courts are patient with relapses and continue to hold the case, provided the defendant returns to treatment. Apparently, research suggests that those with the highest risk of recidivism need a minimum of biweekly status hearings to stay in treatment and drug-free.

Abstinence and continuation in a 12 Step program is the typical treatment model that the courts usually recommend. Some courts try different and innovative treatments where acupuncture is a choice. Others have tried a controlled drinking approach where abstinence is not required as long as the individual carefully controls the amount and use of the substance. This program works best with those who are not heavy substance abusers, although some who like having total control over their own lives may do well with such an approach.

Typically, the defendant is arrested and brought before the magistrate for first appearance within 24 hours. Sometimes the police officer recognizes the defendant from the community and suggests drug court if she or he knows that it is available. This gets passed on to the Sheriff's deputy in the court, who passes it on to the appropriate authorities. If the defense attorney, prosecutor, or magistrate suggests drug court, and the defendant agrees to volunteer, then he or she can be sent directly there by the magistrate-on-duty. Usually that appearance is sometime that day or shortly afterwards. In some cases, statutes that provide for involuntary hospitalization of the defendant are activated. If the arrest includes more than possession of alcohol or other drugs, then it is rare that drug court referral will be made. This is especially true if there is any violence involved in the charge or if selling of the drugs is involved. Sometimes it is difficult to tell, especially if there is possession of a large quantity of drugs that indicates that it will be sold rather than used personally.

If these individuals are still intoxicated at the time of arrest, they may be sent to a detoxification center. Sometimes the detoxification is done in the jail's medical center, if medical intervention is available. Other times subjects are sent to a hospital or special facility and then returned to the jail where they may then be transferred into drug court.

Once in drug court, all of the defendant's records usually are available to the judge and attorneys, who all act together rather than in an adversarial manner, with the goal of helping the defendant to become drug-free. Obviously, the goal of the court is to keep the defendant from re-offending. Thus, careful supervision of the defendant is required with frequent appearances scheduled before the court for monitoring of his or her progress. Usually the social workers or case managers from the drug treatment program are also present at these follow-up court times.

The early success of the drug courts, especially when services were available in the community, prompted the development of other types of courts that could deal with those who have specific problems amenable to treatment. The type of treatment that research suggests is most successful is a cognitive-behavioral model where the behavior is treated along with the mental state that accompanies it. In some cases, psychopharmacological intervention with medication is also recommended, at least for a while, to help the individual remain free of illegal substances. Those most vulnerable to substance abuse relapse include abused women and those with bipolar disorders, especially when there are no mental health services available to supplement substance abuse programs.

Proper medication for these mental health problems may alleviate the need to use alcohol or other drugs to feel better. During the withdrawal period, benzodiazepines such as Ativan (lorazepam) or Serax (oxazepam), antihypertensives such as Catapress (clonidine), Inderal (propanolol), or Tenex (guanfacine), antihistamines such as Vistaril or Atarax (hydroxyzine), or even anti-psychotics such as Trilaphon (perphenazine) may be used. Many former alcoholics use benzodiazepine medication as a substitute, although its addictive properties may make it difficult to continue it indefinitely because the person habituates to the safe doses. Some have used medications such as Methadone to help heroin addicts safely withdraw from the illegal drug, but this has become controversial due to the addictive properties of the Methadone.

It cannot be emphasized enough that the drug court can be successful only if the community has sufficient treatment facilities to deal with the large numbers of defendants who need services. Usually there need to be several public and private residential facilities, as well as out patient service centers, to deal with people with addictions. It is only recently that these facilities are learning how to work with people who have co-occurring disorders or what is frequently called "dual diagnosis"—that is, people who have a serious or at least diagnosable mental illness along with their substance abuse disorder. In some cases, particularly in women with trauma histories, the alcohol or other drugs are used as self-medication and, without the intervention for trauma symptoms, it is difficult to motivate the person to stop using the substances. Even with the best services available, the success rate in drug courts is around 60%, which demonstrates the promise and the complexity in working with this population.

MENTAL HEALTH COURTS

Although deinstitutionalization of the mentally ill in the 1960s in the United States was designed to give the seriously mentally ill the opportunity for community-based treatment rather than long-term hospitalization, the lack of consistent services and inability of this population to follow through with services without closely supervised case management has marginalized this population rather than giving them greater autonomy over their lives. Many of them are homeless, poor, without family contacts, and without resources. They have previous diagnoses of schizophrenia, paranoia, bipolar and major depressive disorders. They may have neuropsychological disorders, and they may be HIV positive or have other medical complications. Most of them have experienced abuse at one or more points in their lives. As a result, jails and prisons have become "de facto hospitals of the last resort" when the severely mentally ill are arrested, usually for non-violent, misdemeanor acts. Unfortunately, the types of intervention that the seriously mentally ill need cannot be provided, so diversion into community-based treatment has been one response. The key, of course, is to be sure that the community can provide adequate intervention

In 2000, the U.S. Congress signed into law P.L. 106–515, legislation that authorized the funding of 100 mental health courts around the country. Other countries have also sent teams of observers to learn about these new demonstration courts in anticipation of developing their own models. NAMI (The National Alliance for the Mentally Ill) can be very helpful in developing peer-support groups and other similar models in communities. The National Mental Health Association has also made it clear that, without protection for the civil rights of those who use the mental health court, it can result in undesirable forced treatment, thus negating the intent of the mental health court to provide intervention in the least restrictive environment possible. While it is too early to tell if the mental health court will keep the mentally ill out of jail and prison, it is believed that the key to success is the availability of intensive casework provided by the court, frequent status hearings such as was suggested by drug court models, and user-friendly, easily accessible resources and other services in the community.

DOMESTIC VIOLENCE COURTS

Another popular problem-solving court is the domestic violence court where perpetrators of domestic violence are deferred into offender-specific treatment programs, either pre or post adjudication. This court was developed with consultation from battered women advocates who learned that many women who refused to testify against their batterers wanted them to get treatment to stop the abuse rather than go to jail or prison. In some cases where the risk of repeated violence was high, court orders for perpetrators to stay away from victims may be accompanied by electronic monitoring with ankle bracelets similar to those used for others on home release programs.

Law enforcement officers have been trained to deal with domestic violence disputes in ways different from those previously suggested. For example, officers are trained to respond in pairs so they can separate the couple and interview each party separately. If there is *probable cause* (the legal standard) to believe that the man is abusing the woman, then the officers are empowered to make an arrest immediately and transport the defendant to jail. Today, all law enforcement officers are made aware of the special danger that can exist when responding to a domestic violence call, while being trained at the Police Academy and during roll calls. Sometimes the abuser is still battering the victim when the officers get to the house or other location. Other times, the situation has already calmed down, and the officers have difficulty in deciding who was the perpetrator.

In some cases, the man quiets down and is quite responsive to the officer, while the woman is still agitated and angry, sometimes even screaming and yelling at the officer. In these cases, it is tempting to arrest them both, especially if the man as well as the woman has physical marks on his body evidencing the woman's aggression against him. Although initially it may be difficult to sort out who is the aggressor, most of the time it is the man who is violent. It is important to remember that, if the woman does use defensive aggression and then is arrested, she may plead guilty just to get released in time to prevent her children from going into foster care. She still is the victim and not the aggressor. These facts come out in the treatment programs that are offered on the other end of the process, but can be devastating in a custody case if officials later decide to terminate their parent-child relationship.

The typical model is to arrest the perpetrator, usually the man, for domestic violence if the law enforcement officer has *probable cause* to make that arrest. This means that the law enforcement officer believes that domestic violence did occur and that the person arrested was the perpetrator. It is on that officer's sworn statement that the arrest goes forward. No longer does a victim have to sign a complaint which, of course, makes it less dangerous for her, but also prevents her from being able to *drop the charges* which was so common in domestic violence cases prior to the new 'pro-arrest' laws.

Once the arrest is made, in the model suggested, the perpetrator is placed in detention to wait for the next regularly scheduled domestic violence court session. In most jurisdictions, this is later in the day, usually within 12 to 24 hours after the arrest. On weekends, it might be longer since domestic violence arrests should have been taken off the bonding schedule. Research has shown that the wait in jail is a helpful deterrent for some perpetrators, particularly those who have never had contact with the criminal justice system previously. Unfortunately, it may make the abuser without any ties to the community even angrier. Now that domestic violence courts have been operational in some jurisdictions for twenty years or more, it is clear that different batterers need different types of intervention.

Once before the judge, the perpetrator has the option of pleading guilty or no-contest (which is treated as a guilty plea) and agreeing to go into a special *offender-specific treatment program*. Like the drug court treatment, the domestic violence treatment program is cognitive-behavioral with an emphasis on changing attitudes and behaviors towards women. However, treatment is mandated here and not voluntary, due to public and domestic safety concerns. If the batterer does not attend the treatment program, then he is sentenced to jail or prison. Often the treatment program is offered by the local battered woman's shelter, but in another location so that the perpetrators and victims are not forced to see each other, either intentionally or accidentally. One of the most popular models is called the "Duluth Model" because it originated in Duluth, Minnesota. However, this model is more psychoeducational rather than therapeutic for abusers, making it difficult, if not impossible, for those perpetrators with mental illnesses to receive effective intervention.

The court monitors the defendant's progress in the treatment program through the use of special probation officers who have direct contact with the counselors who run the treatment program. The research suggests that approximately 25% of the batterers who attend a treatment program (and some research suggests that less than 10% of all batterers ever get to attend the program) will stop their physical and psychological abuse of the victim, 50% will stop their physical abuse, but continue their psychological abuse, and 25% continue to physically and psychologically abuse the victim even while attending the treatment program. There are no data on the cessation of sexual abuse unless the offender is also sent to a special sex offenders' program, which is rare in domestic violence cases. However, there may also be concomitant treatment in drug court programs if alcohol or other drugs were found at the domestic violence site.

These treatment programs are unique in several ways. First, there is no promise of confidentiality, nor does the defendant have *privilege*, which is accorded to others who seek mental health treatment. This means that the treatment provider must communicate information about the treatment to the court, usually on a regular basis. Most important is attendance at the program since it is still difficult to measure whether or not the actual program is successful in changing attitudes, values, thoughts, feelings, and behavior other than reoffenses. Less than 50% of those who are court-ordered into treatment actually attend groups.

Second, the treatment provider may not be well trained in other issues besides domestic violence or drug abuse. Unlike psychologists and other doctoral level mental health professionals who are trained in the broad spectrum of human behavior, both abnormal and normal, these providers are trained only in the specific program to be administered. If the individual is unique in any way, the program may not be tailored to fit, perhaps making it inappropriate for that particular defendant. Thirdly, the treatment program, which is often a psychoeducational model, may not be able to deal with any mental illness or other problem that the defendant demonstrates and, thus, is insufficient to stop all violent behavior. Even so, there is a lot of support for these domestic violence offender-specific treatment programs, especially from victims who believe that the batterer may well stop his violent behavior once he is in a special treatment program. Unfortunately, this does not appear to be the case, but it may well be important to try in order for victims to be willing to take the next steps in order to insure their safety and that of their children.

INVOLUNTARY CIVIL COMMITMENT

Although a part of the civil laws and not criminal law, each state has civil commitment laws or the "hold and treat laws" that permit the involuntary arrest by a law enforcement officer and remand to a crisis center or hospital for those who are deemed mentally ill and dangerous to themselves or others. In most states, these civil commitment laws also include as part of dangerousness that these persons are so mentally ill that they are unable to care for themselves. An attorney is provided for individuals who are arrested, primarily because they are considered so mentally ill as to not be able to properly protect their civil rights and liberty. Taking away someone's liberty is considered a serious act and one that must be done only after careful study and evidence. In most states that have civil commitment statutes, these persons must demonstrate dangerousness—it is not sufficient just to be seriously mentally ill—in order to trigger the act. Further, it is not appropriate to commit those who have only dementia unless they are also demonstrating symptoms of serious mental illness and they are dangerous to themselves and others. There was a time when it was believed that people with dementia could not respond to mental health treatment, but, today, sometimes medication and/or behavior modification may assist in gaining more socially appropriate behavior, even though the dementia is not cured. A guardian may have to be appointed to make decisions about someone with middle or late stage dementia, and usually a nursing home type of care is provided.

In order to hospitalize someone involuntarily, it is typical for law enforcement officers to take the individual to a receiving hospital in their area. There the doctor in charge in the emergency room makes the determination if a 72-hour hold (the usual amount of time given to the doctor to make such a determination) is required or if the patient can be released safely back into the community. Sometimes, a family member just wants to get an agitated or angry patient out of the house, and once he or she calms down, it is apparent that there is no need to detain that person any longer since he or she is no longer dangerous. If there are no records available and no one other than the patient to provide information about history, it is possible that mistakes are made. However, personnel are trained to make these kinds of distinctions and, if there is a question, to err on the side of caution to protect the person and the public. If no crime was committed, then the civil commitment statute is invoked; if a crime has been committed, then the decision is made by the officer whether to arrest and take the person to jail or go directly to the receiving center. Often this decision is made based on the person's behavior—if he or she is still exhibiting extreme aggression, it is safest to take her or him to a receiving center for crisis management—which is usually a dose of anti-psychotic medicine.

In civil commitments, within the 72-hour period (often it is up to a week because the hearings are held only weekly in most jurisdictions), there is a hearing before a magistrate or judge who makes a decision based on evidence whether to hold the person for up to thirty days for treatment or to release the person back into the community as stabilized. These hearings are usually held at the hospital so the severely ill patients do not have to be transported to the courtroom where they might not be able to control their behavior. Psychiatrists and psychologists from the hospital unit may testify as to their recommendations, and the attorney for the individual may also provide psychological testimony by privately hired mental health professionals should there be disagreements. The goal should be the *least restrictive environment* in order for the person to be restored to competency.

If there is need for more than 30-day treatment, then the individual may be sent to the state hospital for long-term treatment. If there is a pending charge, and the individual is deemed *not competent to stand trial*, then the court may order *competency restoration* programs as part of the treatment. This is controversial since many believe that competency restoration programs simply help patients to memorize the roles of the various actors in the court proceedings, but not really to understand the consequences of what may happen to them. In cases where competency cannot be restored within the specified time (usually five years), then charges may be dropped, and individuals may be released if they are no longer a danger to themselves or others. However, this means that the individuals may not get appropriate treatment once they are released. Only the judge can order the release, and it is not automatic but, rather, often based on the seriousness of the crime.

If individuals are still dangerous, then a civil commitment may be reapplied for and obtained for an indefinite amount of time. In the new civil commitment statutes for sex predators, it is an indefinite hold until such time as treatment renders individuals no longer a dangerous sex predator. Obviously, few will ever be released under these strict rules.

One of the most famous cases is that of John Hinkley who has spent the last 20+ years in St. Elizabeth's Hospital, with doctors still arguing if it was his psychotic disorder or a personality disorder that motivated him to shoot at President Reagan, Press Secretary James Brady, and the Washington, D.C. police officer, Thomas Delahante in 1982. In late 2005, Hinkley's treating psychiatrist and his attorneys won him overnight visitation with his parents after a lengthy battle for him to be able to leave the hospital for more than a few hours.

Competency Restoration intervention usually consists of medication plus some group skills training. State forensic hospitals use a fairly routine group treatment approach with all *incompetent-to-proceed (ITP)* defendants. Although there is an attempt to use the newer materials that were developed by the *MacArthur Foundation* project's research on competency and dangerousness, many defendants are unable to follow them. Some develop the ability to simply recite the *Dusky criteria* (see Box 11.2 for synopsis of the case) but do not actually *know* or understand what they mean. Even when they can describe the court proceedings and players involved, they may be so mentally ill that they cannot properly assist their attorneys at trial, and, thus, remain incompetent-to-proceed to trial according to criteria demanded by the statute and hospital staff.

INVOLUNTARY SEX PREDATOR CIVIL COMMITMENT

New case law based on U.S. Supreme Court cases such as *Kansas vs. Hendricks* (1997) and *Kansas vs. Crane* (2002) has supported state laws requiring those defendants convicted of sexual crimes that are deemed to still be dangerous, often classified as sexual predators, to be civilly committed to special treatment centers rather than released into the community after they serve their prison terms. Although challenged as unconstitutional because it is double jeopardy or punishment twice for the same criminal act, the U.S. Supreme Court has ruled that issues of

BOX 11.2

U.S. Case Law that Regulates Intervention with Mentally Ill Defendants

Wyatt v. Stickney	First Federal case that gave specific details to "right-to-treatment" and described the need for individualized treatment programs, staff-patient ratios, etc.
Rouse v. Cameron	First major right-to-treatment case that described the right to treatment as a constitutional right.
Lessard v. Schmidt	First major case that defined previous criteria for Involuntary commitment as "unconstitutionally vague" and put forward "danger to self or others" as the criterion.
Dusky v. U.S.	First U.S. Supreme Court case to define "Competency to stand trial" as factual and rational understanding and ability to assist counsel.
Jackson v. Indiana	Held that it was unconstitutional to confine a mentally incompetent defendant indefinitely. The state must hold the defendant only long enough to determine if competency can be restored in the foreseeable future and, if not, then the defendant must be released or civilly committed.
Donaldson v. O'Connor	U.S. Supreme Court declared that it is unconstitutional to confine non-dangerous mentally ill individual without providing treatment.
Rogers v. Okin, Mills v. Rogers	Patient has the right to refuse medication. However, this right can be overridden if the person is a danger to him- or her-self or others. Patient has right to a full judicial hearing to determine if he or she can refuse the medicine.
Rennie v. Klein	Patient has the right to refuse medication unless a danger to him- or her-self or others but does not have the right to a full judicial hearing. Rather, the determination can be made informally at the hospital.
Youngberg v. Romero	This case extended the right to treatment to developmentally disabled persons.
Harper v. Washington	Prison inmates may have right to refuse medication if not a danger to self or others, but determination can be made at the prison without a full judicial hearing.
Riggins v. Nevada	Pretrial defendant on medication has the right to refuse the medication unless a danger to him or her self or others. The probability that the defendant might become incompetent again is not sufficient to justify forced medication.
Sell v. U.S.	U.S. Supreme Court said that a defendant can only be forced to take medication if it is "medically indicated" and the person is a "danger" and not for other reasons including competency restoration.

public safety make it imperative that these people not be released until they are no longer dangerous. Assessment of the risk of dangerous behavior for those with a history of sexual crimes is quite difficult, especially for those who have not been in the general population for long periods of time as is typical for these prisoners. Treatment programs are not well conceived, staffed, or funded, so the probability that any of those who are sent to sex predator centers will ever be released is quite slim. The court has required psychologists to perform an evaluation and has permitted a civil trial by jury if the prisoner challenges the commitment, but few are won given the fears of the general public, especially if children were the focus of the predatory acts.

INSANITY DEFENSES

Although not exactly a problem-solving court action, most legal systems permit the transfer of defendants who cannot be held responsible for their actions to state facilities for the criminally insane. The concept of *insanity* is one derived by the legal system and not the mental health field. Thus, definitions of what it means to be *insane* are not as precise as are diagnosable mental illnesses and disorders. Not only must someone have a mental illness or disorder, but it must negatively impact on the person's cognitive state of mind and sometimes behavior. Most jurisdictions use a strict cognitive test for insanity today that is often called the *M'Naughten* rule, so-named for a famous 1843 case in England. According to M'Naughten, the defendant must be unable to know the difference between right and wrong or the consequences of his or her behavior. At earlier times, particularly prior to the 1981 attempted assassination of President Reagan by John Hinckley, definitions of insanity created by teams of legal and mental health scholars were used, often permitting the inability to control one's behavior to serve as a component of the defense.

Those defendants who are found *not-guilty-by-reason-of-insanity (NGRI)*, less than 5% of all criminal cases, are usually sent to the state hospital facility for an indefinite period of time. Despite the average person's belief that these people "get away with their crimes," studies show that they are held longer in the hospital than they would have been if they had been sentenced to prison. In fact, most defendants do not want to plead NGRI because they understand they will lose the civil rights that other prisoners have won in the courts as described in Box 11.2. Medication is more likely to be forced, and whatever treatment is available may also not be voluntary. Nonetheless, the inability of jurors to understand and convict on an insanity defense remains one of the problems with the high numbers of mentally ill who end up in prison rather than in the hospital for treatment.

An alternative that some states have turned to is the *Guilty-but-Mentally Ill* defense which, if successful, sends the defendant to the hospital to be treated and then back to prison to serve out his or her sentence. This defense is problematic under the criminal justice system that excuses the mentally ill for their behavior because it is still punishment for actions that they may not be able to control. However, it does solve the problem of public safety while removing mentally ill prisoners from society and theoretically providing them with appropriate treatment.

Finally, the numbers of mentally ill and disordered in jails and prisons have made them de facto mental hospitals without adequate resources for treatment, thus contributing to the high recidivism rate once these people are released. Attempts to provide treatment, avoid punishment of the mentally ill for behavior they cannot control, lower recidivism, and provide for public safety have stimulated the growth of problem-solving courts often called *therapeutic jurisprudence* or *restorative justice*. The most common courts today include drug court, mental health court, (See Box 11.3 for a description on one such court) and domestic violence court. These courts must provide frequent status hearings, intensive case management services, and an array of services easily available for this population in the community in order to be successful.

Women defendants who may find themselves arrested and deferred into any of these courts often need the services of all of them because they tend to be abuse victims who are mentally ill and have substance abuse problems. In addition, they may have child raising problems and few family contacts, and need housing. Special intervention programs for women with co-occurring disorders are now available in some communities. Although women are more likely to volunteer to be deferred into these special courts, they also are more likely to make use of the services if available.

Intervention programs exist for defendants who are declared incompetent-to-proceed to trial because they do not meet the Dusky standards that include factual and rational understanding of the legal system and ability to rationally assist their attorneys in the preparation of a defense. These programs, called Competency Restoration Programs, are usually offered in the hospitals and outpatient facilities if the defendant is deemed not to be dangerous. If they cannot be restored to competency after a certain period of time, usually 5 years for misdemeanor acts and 7 years for non-violent felonies, then they may be released into the community, provided public safety needs are met.

Those convicted of a sexual offense and defined as sexual predators under the law may be sent to a special treatment facility after they serve their prison term. They do have the right to a trial if they protest this civil commitment for an indefinite time period until they are deemed no longer to be a public safety risk. Few of these treatment centers have empirically supported treatment models so, in fact, these laws may well

Model Mental Health Court

Broward County, Florida was the first community in the United States to set aside a therapeutic court that was dedicated to working with the seriously mentally ill who are arrested, usually for non-violent misdemeanor crimes such as shoplifting, loitering, intoxication in a public case, minor theft and robbery, and the like. These people are often floridly psychotic at the time of their arrest. Sometimes they are also intoxicated or high on street drugs, masking their serious mental illness. A community task force decided to try this new therapeutic court after several high publicity cases where poor, mentally ill defendants spent long periods of time incarcerated in jail awaiting hearings on minor charges. In Florida, it is possible to hold a defendant for up to twenty-one days without filing formal charges—and an extra week might be granted if the prosecutor requests it. Determining that it would better serve the community interests to rehabilitate by mental health treatment rather than incarcerate and punish these defendants, a judge with considerable training in mental health treatment volunteered and was assigned to the court, along with representatives from the local mental health community. Students from the doctoral psychology program studying forensic psychology also were available in the court to assist the judge in making appropriate referrals.

Like the other therapeutic courts, the assignment into the correct court often occurs during first appearance, which, in Florida, occurs before a magistrate. During the first five years of the court's history, doctoral students, called interns in the system, screened all those arrested, looking for mental health disorders in the new arrestees. If they were found, and the defendant agreed to volunteer for the mental health court, then the intern testified before the magistrate-on-duty to justify the referral to the mental health court. It was unusual for the magistrate not to make the referral unless there were other records not available to the intern, who was in another building from the magistrate and the attorneys, and appeared with the defendant via closed-circuit television. Other witnesses and other court and mental health records may have been available to the judge, but not yet sent over to the jail.

Once the referral was made, the defendant was brought to mental health court later that day. Sometimes there was difficulty if the defendant was eligible to bond out or the charges were fulfilled by the time-served by the defendant prior to the first appearance in front of the magistrate. A conflict between the therapeutic need for the defendant to obtain treatment and the court's need to discharge the case could occur, and it was usually the defendants' right to make the final decision. Sometimes the defendants were so psychotic and dangerous to themselves that they had to be involuntarily hospitalized to be stabilized. This most frequently occurred when they either forgot or purposely did not take their medication and then got into trouble and were arrested.

Treatment is provided by others in the community, although it is clear that the

---

be a back door into a life sentence for sexual predators, especially those who are known to molest and abuse children.

Insanity statutes permit defendants who commit what would otherwise be called a criminal act to be sent to the hospital for an indefinite period in order to receive treatment for their mental illness. Despite the fears of the general population, rarely are those excused by a successful Not Guilty by Reason of Insanity defense released sooner than their jail or prison sentence would have required.

resources for treating the seriously mentally ill are quite limited. Most of the time the seriously mentally ill need intensive case-work so that their many different needs are well-coordinated. For example, they probably need medication to stabilize them, but, first, they need comprehensive psychological and neuropsychological evaluations to evaluate what medications might be the most useful in reducing symptomology. In many cases, if the right medication is found, individuals are able to stop substance abuse that is related to their search for the right medication. If they continue to abuse substances, then a separate drug program might be recommended. Housing is often a major issue for this population, so case managers need to be familiar with obtaining federal, state, and local housing grants for them. Often they are eligible for Medicare or Medicaid benefits and need assistance in obtaining them. Day treatment centers are also an important option, especially for women who are at high risk for further abuse either at home or on the streets. Many of these women have young children who are in the custody of the Department of Children and Families. It is important to provide intervention so that these women can better parent their children and prevent the cycle of abuse from one generation to another that is so often seen in the criminal justice system.

Approximately 25% of the caseload in mental health court are women, which is an overrepresentation in the criminal justice system where women are less than 10% of the total national criminal justice population. In Broward County, approximately 20% have had between one to nine prior arrests for misdemeanor and 10% have had prior felony arrests. Approximately one-third have had between one to nine prior hospitalizations for mental health problems, while almost one-quarter reported no prior mental health treatment. The most common diagnoses were schizophrenia, bi-polar disorder, major depression, and schizoaffective disorder.

Considering the fact that there are two to ten people referred for mental health court per day in Broward County alone, and as is seen in Box 11.1b, for every two people who volunteer to be deferred into the specialty court, eight others refuse; it is important for law enforcement officers to be aware of these mentally ill people and the resources available for them, if any, in their communities. The goal, of course, is to keep mentally ill people out of jail, but also to get them proper treatment. In some cases, someone who is mentally ill is hassled by the police, becomes agitated, and begins to fight back against the officer, resulting in charges of battery against a law enforcement officer. This could be avoided if that officer is made aware of how to diagnose and deal with seriously mentally ill persons who may be responding more to internal stimuli in their heads rather than what is actually going on in the real world at the moment. Time and patience may be what is needed here.

SUGGESTED READINGS

Berman, G. & Feinblatt, J. (2005). *God courts: The case for problem-solving justice.* Center for Innovation. Delmar, NY: National GAINS Center.

GAINS Center (1999). *Drug courts as a partner in mental health and co-occurring substance abuse disorders diversion programs.* Delmar, NY: National GAINS Center.

Goldkamp, J. D. & Irons-Guynn, C. (2000). *Emerging judicial strategies for the mentally ill in the criminal caseload: Mental health courts in Fort*

Lauderdale, Seattle, San Bernadino, & Anchorage. Washington, DC: U.S. Department of Justice, Office of Justice Programs, Bureau of Justice Assistance. Monograph Pub No. NIJ 182504.

Griffin, P., Steadman, H. J., & Petrilla, J. (2002). The use of criminal charges and sanctions in mental health court. *Psychiatric Services, 53* (10), 1285–1289.

Hills, H. A. (2004). *The special needs of women with co-occurring disorders diverted from the criminal justice system.* Delmar, NY: The National GAINS Center.

Steadman, H. J., Williams Deane, M., Borum, R., & Morrisey, J. P. (2000). Comparing outcomes for major models of police responses to mental health emergencies. *American Journal of Mental Health, 51* (5), 645–649.

CHAPTER 12

Mental Disorders in Youth

Children cope with stress in various ways just like adults. Often they do not share their feelings with the adults in their lives because they see how upset the adults are and do not want to upset them further. Therefore, it is up to the adults to help children get through any stressful situation rather than expect the children to ask for what they need. This means understanding where children are developmentally, understanding their general developmental needs, and at the same time, learning about the individual child's needs. To do this, it is important to know how to recognize the children who have developmental disorders and other mental health problems, the family dynamics in which the child has lived, what kinds of treatment are available for children, and how these factors impact on children who come to the attention of the juvenile justice system. Box 12.1 describes the impact of trauma on a child who experienced the recent Tsunami in Asia in 2004. In this story, it is apparent that the child appeared to have been in what some call "shock" or experiencing an Acute Stress Disorder. The workers who found him used other children to help Jamie find his voice so he could disclose enough information to find his family. Jamie had a supportive family who was able to help him heal and thrive developmentally. There are still many children who are lost whose families perished in the floods that followed that disaster.

In the second story, shown in Box 12.2, Abdul who was older than Jamie, experienced the horrors of war. His parents were not killed but he witnessed others being killed, raped, and tortured. Even after his family was safe and living in another country, Abdul was unable to regain what he had lost during that trauma. Unless there is some way to jump start his own production of the hormone needed for his physical growth, he will remain the physical size of an 8 year old while intellectually and emotionally at his normal developmental age. Others have told stories of children whose hair turns white after experiencing a trauma, probably because their Autonomic Nervous System's fear response stops other biochemicals from necessary production.

BOX 12.1

Children and Trauma: Jamie

Jamie was found wandering around in the streets of a resort town after the Tsunami had swept away his entire family and the hotel in which they were vacationing. He was totally expressionless, did not speak or even whimper, and looked hungry and tired. He stood nearby several rescuers who were digging out the rubble that was left behind and appeared to be watching them. When they stopped digging for a moment, one of the men turned to the child and tried to engage him in conversation. He said nothing but one word, "Jamie". The four men stopped their work and tried to engage the child. One man offered him a half of his own food and Jamie, who they had affectionately named the child, eagerly accepted it, chewing and swallowing it rapidly. He also drank the tea he was offered quickly, too. Jamie was a blonde haired, blue eyed child of about four years of age who was lost in a town where dark haired, brown eyed Asian children lived. One of the men thought to take him to a school where there were other children who looked about his age. Immediately, the children swarmed around Jamie, asking him all kinds of questions in a language that the child did not understand. The police were called and they took him to the hospital to make sure he was not physically hurt and then contacted the coordinators of the relief effort to find out what to do. Quickly, the answer came suggesting that they keep Jamie in the town for a few days to see if anyone else from his family was spared and came looking for him. One of the men, who had a four year old child of his own, took Jamie home to his family.

Although unable to converse with them, Jamie was able to play with the other children in that family and through play began to smile and even laugh again. It was discovered that he was from England and within a few days, members of his extended family, who were located by matching those looking for survivors, came to take him back to his home. Later it was learned that his parents, with whom he was on a vacation were killed in the Tsunami, but somehow, Jamie had the ability to survive. This story was reported by the media with a demonstration of how resilient Jamie was by video taping him laughing and playing with other children, hugging his aunt and uncle who were raising him, and in all ways appearing to be a normal five year old.

Whether Jamie will need further assistance in coping with any residual effects of both losing his parents and having gone through the horrible Tsunami experience alone will remain to be seen. Psychologist Annette LoGrecco, at the University of Miami, has spent the past 15 years researching the effects of such overwhelming trauma on the children who experienced Hurricane Andrew, a major destructive hurricane in South Florida, in 1991. She has found that these children do develop PTSD which leaves them more vulnerable to redevelopment when experiencing new traumas. She has developed various strategies to assist parents and family members in helping these children cope. One of the most important strategies is to assist the family in becoming attached again as they might also become detached from people in struggling to cope with their own reaction to the crisis in their lives.

The children described in these two stories were both said to be developing in a normal and healthy way prior to experiencing the trauma. What about children who are already developmentally compromised in some way. The impact of mental disorders on children has been discussed in earlier chapters addressing serious psychological disorders. This chapter will focus on disorders specific to children, such as developmental disorders and those that impact on children who are seen in the juvenile justice system.

BOX 12.2

Children & Trauma: Abdul

Abdul was 8 years old when his family was living in Kuwait where his father worked in the oil fields. Suddenly, a major war conflict broke out in the streets and all the Palestinian workers were ordered by the Palestine Authority to move to Jordan. Abdul saw people being shot and killed, trampled on by others, and was exposed to the other horrors of war. Although his family was spared, the images were seared in Abdul's brain and he could not erase them. For several months, he was mute, unable to speak to anyone. His family soon settled down to a comfortable existence in a small town near Petra, Jordan where many tourists come to see the lost city found in the early 20th Century. He began to speak again but although Abdul's cognitive and emotional development continued on schedule, he stopped growing physically. At age 13 he was still the size that he was when he was eight years old. His father took him to the doctors in the village in which they lived who recommended doctors in Amman where they made the six to eight hour trip several times. All the doctors said there was nothing physically wrong with Abdul, but he had stopped producing the necessary growth hormone during the time he had the Acute Stress Reaction and nothing they had done for him could make his body produce the hormone again.

DEVELOPMENTAL DISORDERS

When most people hold their baby in their arms for the first time, they check to make sure that he or she has all the right body parts and, as extra assurance, may even count the number of fingers and toes. Unfortunately, it is not so simple to check for disorders of the brain since those often do not become visible until the infant begins to walk and talk. Usually, the first sign that something is wrong comes when there are delays in the development of behavior and cognition. In some rare cases, there is trauma at or close to birth that causes problems with the development of the brain and nervous system, such as a stroke causing damage to blood vessels in a specific area of the brain, premature birth causing incomplete maturation of organs such as the lungs preventing sufficient oxygen to the developing brain, or a metabolic disorder that interferes with the development of the endocrine and digestive systems. There are simple blood tests that can be given when the baby is born to help screen for these types of problems, such as the test for Phenylketonuria (PKU test) that indicates a metabolic problem that may then be corrected.

Sometimes, when the parents know that they both come from families with a history of an otherwise rare genetic disorder or something unusual is noted in the prenatal ultrasound test, they can test a fetus' chromosomes through amniocentesis while it is still in the uterus, and make decisions about whether to continue the pregnancy or how to treat the neonate when it is born. Today it is even possible to perform certain kinds of surgery while the fetus is developing in the uterus. Downs Syndrome, which usually is accompanied by mental retardation, is one of the more common chromosomal abnormalities that can occur,

Table 12.1. Cardinal Signs and Symptoms: Mental Retardation

- IQ below 70
- Deficits or impairments in adaptive functioning
- Communication
- Self care
- Home living
- Social/interpersonal skills
- Self direction
- Academic or work skills
- Health and safety
- Onset before 18 years old

more frequently with pregnancies in older women. Other types of mental retardation can be caused by genetic abnormalities, some of which seem to be found in families or in people who come from a specific region of the world. Since so much of brain development continues after birth until the child is around 20 years old, early identification and intervention in brain disorders may make the difference in how functional the child can become and how the parents learn to cope with the challenges of raising such a child.

Table 12.1 describes the cardinal signs and symptoms of mental retardation that may be seen in seriously developmentally disabled children. These children are afforded special education in their regular schools unless they are so profoundly disabled that they need special care in centers where they may spend the week in residence. Those children with parents who can care for them may take them home for weekends or other special visits. When these children experience a trauma their cognitive limitations may make it difficult for them to make sense out of the crisis situation. They may need special attention as was described by crisis workers during the aftermath of Hurricane Katrina. It is often difficult to separate out those children who may act the same but are traumatized from those who have been previously disabled and are traumatized until the crisis is over and the symptoms abate. But for now, let's look at some of the more well known developmental disorders including mental retardation from various causes.

TOXIC SUBSTANCES

Exposure to toxic substances, called terotogens, which cross the placental barrier in the uterus, can damage a child's brain and nervous system. Other toxic substances have a damaging effect on the child's developing brain and nervous system after birth, such as lead-based paint chips peeling from walls and eaten by babies or second hand-smoke in homes where cigarette smoking is common. Poverty contributes to developmental disorders by preventing the brain and nervous system, which continue to develop for many years after birth, from getting the adequate nutrients or oxygen necessary for proper development. We have learned a great deal about how alcohol and other drugs used by the pregnant woman can irreparably damage the brain and developing nervous system of the fetus, which is why there are warnings placed on many common prescription drugs in addition to warnings to stay away from street drugs and alcohol. Fetal Alcohol Syndrome (FAS) is one of the most serious consequences, and it is often seen in those who are later arrested for impulsive, dangerous, and violent criminal behaviors.

Babies exposed to crack and other cocaine derivatives in utero may also have numerous developmental problems that make them difficult to comfort when they become upset. They are called *inconsolable babies* because they cry constantly no matter what the adults do to try to comfort them. Some of these children never learn how to make themselves feel better or regulate their own emotions, even as adults. They may have speech and language difficulties, including an inability to express themselves accurately. As a result, they have poor social interactions with both peers and adults in their lives. Table 12.2 provides some characteristics which facilitate identification of these babies and children.

Most of the developmental disorders described here cannot be cured because the damaged cells in the brain and nervous system do not re-grow, as do other cells in the body. However, the nervous system does have what we call *plasticity*, or the ability of one cell to adapt to doing the functions of a different cell. The younger the fetus or infant when the damage occurs and the more oxygen and proper nutrients that get to

Table 12.2. Characteristics of Fetal Alcohol Syndrome

- Small for gestational age or in relationship to peers
- Facial abnormalities such as small eye openings
- Poor coordination
- Hyperactive behavior
- Learning disabilities
- Speech and language delays
- Mental retardation or low IQ
- Problems with activities of daily living (ADLs)
- Poor reasoning and judgment skills
- Sleep and sucking disturbances in infancy
- Emotional dysregulation and inconsolability

the developing brain, the more likely that some of the healthy brain cells can take over the role of those that were damaged. Sometimes retraining the brain cells is necessary, and again, the sooner this occurs, the more likely the success. Intervention programs that teach parents how to regulate the behavior and environment of these children can help establish good habits and functional skills despite low cognitive ability. Simple directions, patience, and repetition are important in these programs. Stem cell research is on the frontier of even newer techniques to help the damaged brain and nervous system to learn to function again. But even school-based learning can be helpful, which is one reason why it is best to place developmentally delayed children in intellectually stimulating environments as early as possible.

TOURETTE SYNDROME

Tourette Syndrome is considered both a neurological and psychological disorder that is characterized by sudden, rapid, involuntary movements (tics) and verbalizations (often curse words) that occur frequently throughout the day and worsen when the child is under stress. The tics and other repetitive movements, including vocalizations, often begin when the child is young, sometimes under 5 years old, but usually not later than 18 years old. This is considered evidence that the immature brain has some responsibility in their difficulties with impulse control. Also implicated is an abnormal metabolism of neurotransmitters, particularly dopamine, which controls movements, and serotonin, which controls numerous emotional responses. It is not clearly understood why there is focus on sexual and other inappropriate verbalization and cursing (copralalia) by the child, but some believe that it has something to do with their overwhelming urge to say something that is otherwise "forbidden." There also is a genetic component to this disorder since it is likely to be found in families. Boys have a greater risk of displaying the symptoms.

There is a greater likelihood of children with Tourette Syndrome also developing Attention Deficit Hyperactivity Disorder and Obsessive-Compulsive Disorder, which is sometimes called the triadic disorders because they commonly appear together. Although these children may also have learning problems, they usually have good cognitive skills and intelligence and can learn with special attention. Many Tourette Syndrome children develop sleep disorders which may be related to the serotonin metabolism. Some children with Tourette Syndrome also have a psychotic disorder, but this is rare. Children with Tourette Syndrome do not have any predisposition to aggressive, violent, or criminal behavior, although they may be difficult to deal with should they be in a non-stable environmental crisis situation.

PERVASIVE DEVELOPMENTAL DISORDER (PDD) AND AUTISM SPECTRUM DISORDERS

Today we believe that there is a continuum of mental disorders that are caused by both deficits in the brain development and severe emotional dysregulation that interferes with the child's ability to attach and form relationships with adults and peers. It does not necessarily impact on intelligence or cognitive abilities, but some of the more severely affected are not able to express their thoughts verbally. These disorders are called *Pervasive Developmental Disorders (PDD)*, and they range in seriousness from those that make it difficult to live a normal life to those that are annoying, allowing the person to function in the world with some assistance. Most of these children are placed on a long list of medications, which by itself indicates just how pervasive are the effects of this disorder on their development and ability to function. Parents are usually offered a support group, and it is widely known clinically that raising a PDD child takes its toll on the parents' marriage and on the emotional health of the entire family.

It is important for First Responders to remember that these children will need special attention if they are in a stressful situation because they cannot reregulate themselves when their environment is unstable. Many of them have been mainstreamed in schools with the addition of a special aide who gives them one-to-one attention all through the day. So, whether it is chaos from living in the New Orleans Superdome with thousands of people after Hurricane Katrina or emotional upset in a home where family members are grieving the death of another member, it must be expected that these children will need extra attention just to get through the crisis situation. They are vulnerable and at risk for a myriad of problems.

Autism Spectrum Disorders

The most common and perhaps the most serious PDD is *autism* and its related disorders. Autistic children have severe communication difficulties in their relationships. They often have difficulties in social or emotional reciprocity with peers and adults, perhaps because they have impaired language and speech. Most autistic children have rigid stereotyped and repetitive behaviors that make them seem odd to other children and adults. Description of the cardinal signs and symptoms in the Autism Spectrum Disorders can be found in Table 12.3 along with the typical regimes needed to manage these children. Most autistic children are placed on several different medications to address various dysfunctional systems in addition to behavioral therapy regimes that appear to be helpful in allowing these children to lead functional lives so the common classes of medications used with children diagnosed with autism is also found in Table 12.3. Autism may negatively impact cognitive

Table 12.3. Cardinal Signs and Symptoms: Autism Spectrum Disorders

- Onset is prior to three years old
- As child gets older there is some improvement but rare for adults to live completely independently
- Delay in language development
- Impaired social interactions
- Inability to use nonverbal social behaviors
- Inability to make friends at own age level
- Inability to share joy or other emotions spontaneously
- Difficulty in initiating conversations
- Idiosyncratic conversations
- Does not use normal social cues for reciprocal interactions
- Lack of spontaneous and creative play at age level

Common Interventions using Medication
- Psychostimulants (ADHD symptoms)
- SSRIs (Perseveration, obsessions, aggression, depression, anxiety)
- Alpha-2 Receptor Agonists & Propranolol (explosive behavior & aggression)
- Mood Stabilizers (aggression & mood lability)
- Opioid Antagonists (Naltrexone for self injurious behaviors, stereotypy)
- Conventional & Atypical antipsychotics (aggression, agitation, self-injury)
- Buspirone (anxiety)
- Anticonvulsants (seizures, aggression, impulse control, mood lability)
- Hormones (melatonin for sleep, glucocorticoids)

functioning as well as social and emotional regulation, so that some children have few resources with which to address this disorder, while others can do much more intellectually, despite their serious limitations in other areas. Raising an autistic child is a challenge for most parents who need to join a support group to help them get through difficult times and share their successes.

Aspergers Disorder

Aspergers Disorder or Syndrome is another PDD that negatively impacts on a child's (or adult's) communication and social relationships with others. However, it is less severe than autism, and the children frequently have higher IQs despite their inability to connect socially with people. If we look back, some very creative people who have seemed odd but talented might now be diagnosed with Aspergers Disorder. Like other PDD children, those with Aspergers Disorder often cannot understand the social cues that others signal to them during an interaction. They become frustrated and may resort to rigid stereotyped patterns of interactions, including strange body movements that resemble tics, but

Table 12.4. Cardinal Signs and Symptoms: Asperger's Disorder

- Develops later than autism or other Pervasive Developmental Disorders
- No delays in language
- No delays in cognitive skills
- Poor use of non-verbal cues of behavior (e.g. body postures, facial expressions, eye connection, body posture, and gestures).
- Impaired social interactions
- Stereotypical and repetitive mannerisms and behaviors
- Motor delays or clumsiness
- Prefer to work alone on own interests than with other people even if they share the same interests
- Engages in rituals and rigid routines
- More restrictive interest areas than Obsessive Compulsive Disorder
- Preoccupation with certain areas, things, or parts of things

often in larger patterns. They may develop an extreme focus in one particular area, often computers or parts of objects. However, they differ from those with more serious disorders in that there is no clinically significant delay in any other areas such as cognitive development or self help skills except for an inability to understand and succeed in social interactions. Table 12.4 lists the cardinal signs and symptoms to diagnose Aspergers Disorder.

ATTENTION DEFICIT DISORDERS

Perhaps the most widely diagnosed mental disorder in children is what is called *Attention Deficit Disorder (ADD)* or *Attention Deficit Hyperactive Disorder* (ADHD). These children are frustrating to be with because they cannot regulate their attention and concentration by themselves, yet in other areas appear quite normal. Those with ADHD do not solely have concentration problems and stare into space, as do those with ADD; they also fidget, move uncontrollably, have repetitive and annoying behaviors, and disrupt others. These children have poorly regulated sleeping and waking patterns, often seen in infancy, but they are not usually seen as problematic until entrance into school where they are expected but unable to conform to the rules and behavioral limits. Although those with ADD or ADHD are usually placed in the mental illness classification, it is thought that there is some form of brain dysfunction that contributes to their causation. Many of these children's problematic behaviors disappear after the brain matures in their late teenage years, which supports the argument in favor of brain dysfunction. If special accommodations are not made for these children, they may fail to learn at their appropriate rate, they may develop socially undesirable habits, they may not learn to regulate their own emotions, and they may not engage in good peer relationships. Today, it is becoming more common to see adults who are diagnosed with ADD or ADHD. Although ADHD is thought to have begun in childhood, it is likely that it was undiagnosed or not properly treated and continued into adulthood.

Although good behavioral control of the environment can help children with these attention deficit disorders learn to function successfully, most people turn to medication as a solution and rarely put the behavioral controls into action because they are difficult to implement. For example, it is important to reduce the stimulation in ADHD children's environment, so that they can focus on one thing at a time. However, other children in the home or classroom can thrive with a lot of stimulation, so this solution accentuates the ADHD child's differences from the others and may negatively impact the child's self-esteem.

It is important to help ADD or ADHD children learn to regulate their own emotions. This takes patience on the part of the parents and teachers and repeated training emphasizing the positive strides the child makes, no matter how small they may be. More often, the child's annoying behaviors are usually attended to, often in a punishing way, so that the child is constantly experiencing negative consequences rather than positive reinforcement. This only makes these children more anxious and lowers their self-esteem so they are less likely to accomplish tasks that they could otherwise easily accomplish. Anxiety disorders may develop in this way. Some of these children are disciplined and placed in time-out, and often they are sent to their rooms that are filled with stimulating materials. All this accomplishes is to remove the annoying child from the parent's presence for a period of time. Instead, a carefully constructed behavioral plan should be followed using rewards generously and punishment only sparingly for gross misbehaviors. Since the ADD or ADHD child cannot follow sequences easily, it is best to work on one or two behaviors at a time, rather than trying unsuccessfully to correct all of them. Table 12.5 lists the cardinal signs and symptoms in the ADD and ADHD child and some of the more common interventions that are utilized.

Medication is often used for these children even though behavioral controls often work equally as well. However, applying behavioral controls take time and energy for parents and teachers which may be unrealistic given the other demands on their time. Stimulants such as Ritalin or Concerta are the most common drugs prescribed. Mood regulators such as lithium-based drugs or those in the Selective Serotonin Reuptake Inhibitor (SSRI) category or those that also regulate norepiniphrine are used when the child also has difficult regulating his or her emotions. Care must be taken when using SSRIs as they both can precipitate a manic disorder which is difficult to diagnose in an already hyperactive child or in older children have been said to precipitate suicidal thoughts and feelings. If the child engages in behavior problems, an anti-convulsant medication used as a mood stabilizer may also be added to the regime. In cases where the child does not tolerate the typical

Table 12.5. Cardinal Signs and Symptoms: Attention Deficit/Hyperactivity Disorder

- Usually detected in elementary school
- More common in boys or girls
- Often has a learning disability
- May develop substance abuse problems
- No attention to details and careless
- Cannot sustain attention
- Fails to listen
- Cannot follow through on instructions
- Organizational difficulties
- Loses things
- Easily distracted
- Forgetful
- Squirms and fidgets in seat
- Runs about and climbs excessively
- Cannot play quietly
- "on the go and driven"
- Excessive talking
- Impulsive

Comprehensive Intervention
- Situational Intervention
  - Involve teacher
  - Involve parents
- Behavior Control
  - Therapist/child set goals
- Psychopharmacology
- Psychostimulants 60–75% effective on symptoms—Cylert less effective (50%)
- If child does not have ADD/ADHD medication may still result in increased attention, decreased motor activity, & improvement on learning tasks.
  - Psychostimulants—FDA Approved Ritalin, Concerta
  - Selective Norepinephrine Reuptake Inhibitor (Strattera; FDA approved)
  - Buproprion
  - Tricyclics
  - Selective Serotonin Reuptake Inhibitors
  - MAOIs
  - Alpha 2 receptor agonists
  - Antipsychotics & atypical antipsychotics

medication regime, a small dose of a drug in the atypical anti-psychotic category may be given because these drugs impact on some of the same neurotransmitters that need to be regulated. It should be emphasized that there has been little research on these medications for children, and, other than the stimulants, most are not approved by the Federal Drug Administration (FDA) for use in children whose brains and nervous systems are still developing.

MENTAL DISORDERS IN CHILDREN

In addition to the developmental disorders described above, children also are known to develop many of the mental disorders that are similar to adults. The most common are Mood Disorders including Depression and Bipolar Disorders, Anxiety Disorders such as Separation Anxiety, Obsessive-Compulsive Disorder, General Anxiety Disorder, and Social Phobia and Schizophrenia. These disorders are described more fully in the earlier chapters. However, in some cases there are intervention and treatment plans that are considered best practices and can be found in Box 12.3.

CHILD ABUSE AND PTSD

Although we discuss PTSD earlier, we will include a discussion of how it manifests itself in children, particularly those who are exposed to child abuse or domestic violence in their homes. Child maltreatment, which encompasses physical and sexual abuse of children, neglect, and other forms of psychological abuse, has been one of the more disturbing causes of PTSD. According to the statistics collected by the U.S. Department of Health and Human Services, over 3 million children are reported abused each year in the United States, with almost one million of the reports substantiated. About 25% of these calls were for physical abuse, and about 15% were for sexual abuse. An additional 12% were for multiple forms of abuse. The rest were for various forms of psychological abuse and neglect. Two-thirds of these children are from Caucasian homes, 30% from African American homes, 13% from Hispanic homes, 1.3% from Pacific Islander/Asian American homes, and 2.5% from American & Alaskan Native homes. Approximately 1200 children each year are killed by abuse, with 80% under the age of five, and almost one-half under the age of one year old.

Although almost two-thirds of the known perpetrators of child abuse are women, over half of them were charged with psychological abuse and neglect. Three-quarters of those who committed child sexual abuse were men. In over 75% of substantiated cases, the perpetrators were the child's parents. Contributing factors included substance abuse, poverty and economic strain, lack of parental skills, and domestic violence. In the United States, the agency that is set up to handle cases of child abuse is in the Department of Health and Human Services. It is usually called Child Protective Services (CPS), although it may vary from state to state with Department of Children and Families (DCF) or Department of Youth and Families (DYFS) also common.

It is mandatory for most human service professionals to report suspected child abuse to the proper authorities in their jurisdiction, usually the local law enforcement or social service agency. The case is then investigated, and there are several possible outcomes. First, the abuse is

---

BOX 12.3

Model Therapeutic Interventions & Treatment

Depression

Psychodynamic Therapy
Cognitive Behavior Therapy
Psychoeducational Intervention
Group Interventions
Interpersonal/Family therapy
Biological
Pharmacotherapy (antidepressants)
Electroconvulsive Therapy (ECT)

Bipolar Disorder

Cognitive Behavioral Therapy
Psychoeducational Interventions
Group Interventions
Interpersonal/Family therapy
Stress Management
Pharmacotherapy (lithium/anticonvulsants)

Psychotic Disorders

Schizophrenia
Individual therapy (play therapy with children)
Family therapy
Behavioral Therapy
Social skills training
Speech and Language therapy
Pharmacotherapy (atypical/conventional antipsychotics)

Anxiety Disorders

Separation Anxiety Disorder
Play Therapy
Sand Tray Therapy
Cognitive Behavioral Therapy (more effective with adolescents)
Systematic Desensitization/Relaxation Training
Family Therapy
Pharmacotherapy (SSRIs, Benzodiazepines)

OCD—comprehensive treatment
Exposure with Response Prevention (ERP)

Cognitive Behavior Therapy
Relaxation Training
Family therapy
Pharmacotherapy (SSRIs, TCAs, benzodiazepines)

GAD—Comprehensive Treatment

Behavior therapy
Cognitive Behavior Therapy
Relaxation training/Stress Management
Psychodynamic Therapy
Psychoeducational intervention
Pharmacotherapy (Benzodiazepines, SSRIs, Buspirone)

Social Phobia

Behavioral interventions
Systematic Desensitization/Relaxation Training
Contingency Management
Modeling
Cognitive Behavior Therapy
Self control/Self instructional training
Rational Emotive Behavior Therapy (REBT)
Pharmacotherapy (SSRI's, Buspirone, Clonidine)

PTSD

Treatment must build:
1. Safety & stabilization
2. Symptom reduction & memory work
3. Developmental skills

Using:

Psychoeducational approaches
Social skills training (Dialectical Behavior Therapy—DBT)
Psychodynamic therapy
Sand Tray Therapy
Cognitive Behavioral Therapy
Trauma Specific therapy
Family Therapy
Pharmacological therapy
Educational assistance
Remedial interventions for developmental disturbances

---

not found and the case is dismissed. Second, it is not possible to decide whether or not the abuse occurred, often because of the age of the child or the inability of the child to communicate accurately, and the case is considered *unfounded* or *unsubstantiated*. This does not mean the abuse did not occur, but, rather that abuse cannot be proven. Third, the abuse is found to be *substantiated*, and the CPS takes jurisdiction of the child for the state. Sometimes the child is placed in a shelter if there is thought to be immediate danger, and the parents are ordered into court for a hearing on what should occur next. Usually the caseworker has developed a treatment plan that the parents must follow before the child is permitted to return home. In other cases, the child is permitted to remain in the parents' home, but the parents must still comply with a treatment plan with supervision or monitoring until it is felt that the child is safe from recurring abuse.

Approximately 15% of children are removed from their families and placed in detention centers or foster homes for a longer time to protect them from further abuse. Social workers who usually work for CPS agencies tend to be overloaded with cases and underpaid for their services. The number of children in foster care keeps rising each year, while the number of licensed foster care homes is shrinking, especially those for emotionally disturbed children. Whenever possible, state agencies try to find relatives where these children can live, called *kinship* care. Although some services are provided for children in foster care, in fact, rarely are they offered therapy specific to the PTSD that they may evidence. More often they are placed on psychotropic drugs and maintained without any serious interventions.

Children spend an average of 3 years in foster care, entering around 8 years old and leaving around 11 years old. Most are reunited with their parents who may or may not have completed their treatment plan. Less than 12% are adopted, and even fewer are formally emancipated, although they may become runaways and not found until they are adults. One-third of those in foster care are indeed teenagers, and when they reach age eighteen, they are cut off from any further services. One study found that half of these 18 year olds were unemployed, one-third did not finish high school despite the fact that 90% were attending prior to being cut off from services, one-third were on some form of public assistance, one-quarter of the males and one sixth of the females were physically assaulted during the first year out of services, and one-fifth were incarcerated within a year. Half could not obtain adequate medical care, and less than half of those who were receiving mental health services prior to termination still could access care during the first year off services. Over 85% of delinquent youth in the detention center in one study and the same percentage in the jails and prisons with PTSD from child abuse give an estimate of the relationship of crime and child abuse. Obviously, these youth need continued care, but they are unable to obtain it once they turn 18 years old.

Girls are more likely than boys to be sexually abused as children, usually by males. Unfortunately, it is more difficult to protect these children, especially if the alleged perpetrator is their father or stepfather. When boys are sexually abused, their perpetrator is also often a male, usually a relative or trusted authority figure. The recent disclosures of the large numbers of priests who were simply transferred to another community after allegations were disclosed of sex abuse of children (or women, for that matter) is a prototype of the difficulties in protecting children. Even when they do disclose, no one wants to believe them, especially if the abuser is a socially skilled offender. Yet, the cost in physical and mental health for these children, all through childhood and adult years, is astronomical. The costs for CPS teams, absenteeism from work, dollars spent for medical and mental health, special education, and crime prevention and recidivism prevention are at an all time high.

There are newer ways to assess for child abuse using both the child's own descriptions within the context of their lives and assessment of impact from trauma using standardized psychological tests. It is important to make sure the child is using language appropriate to her or his developmental age and is free from the coercion of either parent during the disclosure. Often young children make a disclosure and then emotionally shut down and cannot continue repeating their story to others, especially those not trained in questioning children their age or who do not use props that they often need to prompt their re-disclosure. Even teenagers are better able to report more details when allowed to use props such as drawings, puppets, stuffed animals, or even anatomically explicit dolls. Some children feel much better after making the disclosure, while others become even more terrified that the perpetrator will retaliate. Although children are most likely to disclose to a non-offending parent, the courts are reluctant to believe them, making parents less able to protect their own child.

Unfortunately, the courts are unable to assist protective parents in trying to protect their children from abusers without evidence that matches the requirements in whichever type of court the case is heard. In family court, the burden of proof of the evidence is usually *more likely than not* or *preponderance of the evidence*; in juvenile dependency court it is usually *clear and convincing evidence* or around 75%; and in juvenile delinquency or criminal court, it is *beyond a reasonable doubt*. Even more damaging to children is when the court places the child in the home of an alleged offender, sometimes as a punishment to a parent who complains too much or who is accused of coaching the child in order to alienate the other parent in highly contested custody cases. It is important to remember that child abuse investigations can be closed as *unfounded* or *unsubstantiated*, which does not mean that the abuse did not occur, but, rather that it cannot be proven to the evidentiary standard necessary. This often happens with children under the age of five, especially in situations where domestic violence also has occurred and the abuser claims the victim suffers from a very controversial condition called *Parental Alienation Syndrome*. There are no empirical data to support the existence of such a syndrome in children who are hostile towards and refuse to spend time with a parent even though some children do behave in this manner and some parents do engage in behaviors that may appear to have caused the child's alienation or even, disengagement from a parent.

Although reporting child sexual abuse is mandatory for professionals in certain categories including all mental health workers, in fact, reporting it may leave the child less protected than before the report is made. Judges in dependency court send children back to abusive parents in far too many cases. In family court, even if the offending parent does not obtain joint custody of the child, it is likely that he or she will obtain unsupervised visitation or other access. If the offending parent has his or her own therapist, the child may not be believed if abuse reoccurs since the therapist now has a stake in believing the therapy was successful in preventing the offender from further molestation. Rarely does the child who makes the report get adequate psychological support or treatment, making it even more difficult to protect the child. Obviously, our system is not protecting children adequately and may need a complete overhaul.

DOMESTIC VIOLENCE

Children who are exposed to domestic violence are even less protected than those who are physically abused. While child abuse victims usually get some protection from CPS workers and the dependency court judge who has some training, albeit limited, the judge who sits on the family court bench is mostly disinclined to take away an admitted perpetrator's access to his or her children, even when experts testify to the damage noted in the child. If the perpetrator denies the abuse, the judge who is determining child custody and visitation issues is often less prepared to take swift and decisive action to protect the child. Rather, the courts have taken the standard, which is the *best interests of the child* and interpreted it to mean that the child must have an equal relationship with both parents. In fact, in many family courts, the judge appears to give more weight to the parent's right to have access to the child than the child's right to be physically and mentally safe. Domestic violence advocates in most states have lobbied legislators to include a *presumption* that shared parental responsibility is not appropriate (because it is not possible for batterers to share power) when there has been domestic violence in the relationship. However, most state statutes only require judges to take domestic violence into their deliberation, rather than have it be an automatic blocker for shared custody, unless the batterer (who has the burden of proof) is able to prove he no longer will abuse his power, control others or use violence to get his needs met.

Even more detrimental to the child's welfare are the *friendly parent* statutes in many states, where the parent who pretends to be the most accommodating to the other parent is more likely to be awarded custody and more access to the child. It is difficult for a battered woman to be friendly towards the person who abused her, and when she does act friendly, the batterer often takes it as a signal that she wants to reconcile. It is also difficult for a mother to allow the child access to his or her father (men are usually, although not always, the perpetrators of domestic violence, with 95% men to 5% women known to be abusers) when her priority is to protect her child. Unfortunately, these protective mothers are challenged by both their abusers and some other professionals and said to create phony syndromes such as *Parental Alienation Syndrome* or *Psychological Munchausen-by-Proxy*, which occurs when parents are accused of complaining about a child's mental health just to gain attention from mental health experts for themselves, with no empirical data to support their complaints. Nevertheless, it is common to hear lawyers arguing that these syndromes are present, backed up with implausible data from other professionals.

Children exposed to domestic violence or child abuse often are identifiable by the PTSD that they experienced. Table 12.6 has a list of criteria that may be observed in these children at different developmental stages. Common interventions for children with PTSD may be found in Box 12.3 above.

RAPE

Surveys consistently report that approximately 25% of all teenage girls have been sexually assaulted or raped before the age of eighteen. In some cases, girls are raped by boyfriends who do not pay attention to the girl when she wants to stop the kissing and making-out. The old stereotyped jokes about a girl saying "no" until the boy persuades her to say "yes" by his sexual prowess, unfortunately, is still alive and well in many communities. A large percentage of those raped by their dates were given one of the so-called *date-rape* drugs, which, unbeknownst to the young women, was slipped into their drinks at a party. These young women often have drunk alcohol from a common punch bowl (which is illegal in most states, but that doesn't stop teens from drinking alcohol at parties) although some are given the drug at a bar or even at a private club. *Rohypnol* (called *Roofies*), *GHB*, and *Ketamine* are the most common drugs that are used because they are colorless, odorless, and difficult to detect in the blood or urine. The fear and horror that is experienced when the young woman awakens and realizes that she has been raped by one or more young men whom she trusted produces a long lasting trauma response. A description of the problems seen at one campus can be found in Box 12.4

OPPOSITIONAL AND CONDUCT DISORDERS

Children who are persistently oppositional may develop a conduct disorder once they begin school. It is difficult to get these children to respond to discipline because they take every attempt to train them as a challenge to begin another power struggle. Children with Oppositional Defiant Disorder are angry but still engage with the parent or other significant people in their life while those with Conduct Disorder

Table 12.6. PTSD Criteria by Age

Infants (0 to 36 months old)
- Hypervigilance
- Exaggerated startle response
- developmental regressions
- Clinging behavior
- Body dysregulation
- Nightmares
- Delayed speech and language

Pre-School (3 to 5 years)
- Avoidant behavioral symptoms
- Intense attachment problems
- Poor social skills

School Age (5 to 10 years)
- Regression in toilet habits
- Poor language skills
- Ostracism by peers
- Attentional disorders
- School failures
- Less consolidation of memories
- Obsessional retelling of details
- Excessive emotional arousal
- Hyperalertness and fears
- Dangerous behavior
- Sense of a foreshortened future

Adolescents (13 to 16 years old)
- Similar to adult PTSD
- Antisocial behaviors (truancy, stealing, sexual acting out, drugs)
- Dangerous reenactments of trauma
- School failures
- Attentional problems
- Poor peer relationships
- Inconsistent limits and boundaries
- Rage escalates if not permitted contact with peers
- Dissociation from self and community

usually are disengaged from others. Those with Conduct Disorder often have been (or felt) abandoned and many of them have not had to account for their behavior to anyone. These children or youth are exhausting to deal with because they are always feeling that they have

BOX 12.4

Potentially fatal date-rape drugs bring national problem to UW

A few drops. A couple of minutes. That was all it took.

When friends found her, the University of Washington sorority member was passed out on the bathroom floor, barely breathing, her body wracked by convulsions.

What hit the woman was Gamma Hydroxybutyrate, or GHB—a drug with a reputation.

On the all-night rave scene, it's a way to get a drunk-like high without the hangover. At crisis centers, it's a "date-rape" drug. In emergency rooms, it's a potential killer.

In Washington, college counselors, Greek advisers, police detectives and doctors have been on the lookout for GHB and two other powerful drugs—Rohypnol and Ketamine. They are concerned about the sometimes fatal effects of recreational use of the drugs and reports that they've been used to incapacitate women who were then sexually assaulted.

A string of incidents in Seattle this year, including the recent arrest of UW football player Jerramy Stevens on suspicion of drugging and raping a student, has raised fears that a national problem has hit home.

"It wasn't until this year that they hit this campus," said John Rhoades, executive director of the Interfraternity Council at the UW. "Unfortunately, it's also apparently present in our community."

The 22-year-old sorority sister, who asked not to be identified, wasn't raped. She took the drug at the urging of a friend who said it would make her "muscles tingly."

She didn't know that after a night of drinking beer, sampling even a small amount of GHB would trigger a dangerous chain reaction. Her blackout lasted several hours.

"When I woke up in the hospital it was the scariest thing in the world," she said. "I had to consciously think about inhaling and exhaling, and if I didn't, I felt like I was going to die."

On a national level, the drugs have been a concern for nearly a decade. They've been slipped into drinks to chemically knock out victims, often leaving them with no memory of what happened the night before.

Rohypnol, known on the street as "roofies," first showed up along the southern border of the United States in the late 1980s. A decade later, 38 states had reports of sexual assaults involving the drug.

Congress responded by passing a 1996 law that applies harsher penalties to those convicted of distributing Rohypnol to someone without that person's knowledge or consent, and with the intent to commit a violent crime. Rohypnol's use has waned in recent years, but GHB and Ketamine are gaining popularity, authorities say.

GHB has been linked to 65 deaths, including 19 since 1997, according to the U.S. Drug Enforcement Administration. The federal government and 25 states have restricted the use and sale of the drug.

Last year, as abuse of Ketamine soared, the government countered by classifying the anesthetic as a controlled substance.

In Seattle, police are investigating a half-dozen cases of suspected date-rape druggings that have occurred since January. Three of them, including the Stevens case, are related to UW fraternity parties.

Evidence hard to find

All of the victims suspect they were slipped drugs in cups of punch or open beverage containers, said Lt. Neil Low of the Seattle Police Department's Special Assault Unit.

"It's not like it's happening at wedding receptions," Low said. "It's at a getting-to-know-you-type party . . . Beer blasts, that type of thing."

In King County, police have yet to document the use of a date-rape drug in any sexual assault, Low said. Across the country, collecting scientific evidence that women who were raped had been slipped these drugs has proven extraordinarily difficult.

The drugs move through the body quickly. Standard screenings in hospitals

BOX 12.4 (Continued)

are unlikely to pick up these particular drugs. And because the drugs can make the victim black out, it often takes awhile for women to piece together what happened, delaying necessary tests.

The alleged drugging in the Stevens case happened at a party June 3 at the Sigma Chi fraternity house near the UW campus, police say.

The end-of-the-year "Jacked Up" bash drew a big crowd that included Stevens and a 19-year-old female freshman. Stevens and the victim are acquaintances and talked at the party. The woman's friends said Stevens was "coming on" to her.

The woman later told police she had five beers over the course of the evening. One of the beers, she said, was already open when someone handed it to her. It didn't take long for the woman to feel the effects. Her friends said she was "unable to keep her balance" and acted as if "she was drugged."

When the friends took her back to her sorority house around 1:30 a.m., they said they ran into Stevens and another UW football player. They were in the alley that connects Sigma Chi with the sorority.

The friends dropped the victim off at the front door. About two hours later, a UW student called 911 and reported a possible rape in progress. Police responded but didn't find the two people described by the witness.

The woman woke later that morning with no memory of what happened the night before or how she got home.

She was in her room, dressed only in her T-shirt and her bra, which was scrunched down around her waist. The fleece jacket Stevens was wearing the night before was in her room, she told detectives.

Police are still investigating. Stevens, who denies attacking the woman, has not been charged with any crime.

Sororities take precautions

Date-rape drug fears have prompted some UW sororities to take extra safety measures.

Mahsa Yeganeh said that in addition to Interfraternity Council- and Panhellenic-sponsored workshops, her sorority, Chi Omega, incorporates discussions about rape and assault prevention into their pledge-education program.

"We have discussions with our new members about what's safe," Yeganeh, a junior, said. "We tell them, 'Don't pick up a drink if you don't know what's in it, and always get your own drinks.' We always travel in groups of two or three, and we never leave a girl at a house alone."

For Yeganeh, the threat of date-rape drugs is real. A close friend believes she was slipped something in a bar in Mexico. She was lucky. When she passed out, friends were there to take her to the hospital.

Katie Smith, a UW senior who is also in a sorority, works with the university Committee on Alcohol and Substance Awareness, which offers presentations to fraternities and sororities.

"Just to be knowledgeable about what's out there is really important," Smith said.

Date-rape drugs do come up in the discussions, Smith said, but she personally views situations like the alleged drugging and rape in the Stevens case as isolated incidents.

"The majority of guys who live around here are really great guys," she said.

For at least five years, most college campuses have offered educational presentations and included drugs such as

been cheated or that they are being picked on unfairly. Yet, they do not understand how to actually read the social cues from others, so people do shy away from them.

Many of those declared delinquent have had conduct disorders from the time they were very young. If they continue to display anti-social

Rohypnol and GHB in literature about date rape.

In 1997, the Rape Treatment Center at Santa Monica/UCLA Medical Center introduced a national campaign at a news conference attended by Attorney General Janet Reno.

Through a partnership with the national Interfraternity Council, the center made videotapes available to fraternities and sororities across the country. The public service announcement they created took an unusual approach; it tells men that administering these drugs can be fatal.

"These are very dangerous weapons; these drugs—you can kill someone," said Gail Abarbanel, founder and director of the Rape Treatment Center. "They're just as dangerous as a gun or a knife, particularly when they're mixed with alcohol."

Many colleges give female students lists of ways to protect themselves—by not accepting open beers or drinks in open containers, for example. But many also focus on encouraging students to look out for their friends.

"A lot of times if they see a peer who appears to be drunk, their response is let the person sleep it off," Abarbanel said. "But in these cases it's really a medical emergency. You need to call 911."

Better testing needed

Getting a handle on the extent of the problem is nearly impossible, for a number of reasons.

Date rape is underreported in general, experts say. And testing for drugs such as Rohypnol and GHB has proven difficult—both because of how quickly they go through the victim's system and because it took awhile for agencies to hone proper procedures for testing.

The Washington State Toxicology Lab established an in-state testing center for date-rape drugs about 18 months ago and has been sending recommended protocols for collecting samples to hospitals and agencies that work with rape victims.

"I guess it all began because a lot of hospitals were wanting their samples tested for date-rape drugs and there was really nowhere to send them," said Fiona Couper, a senior fellow at the Washington State Toxicology Lab.

Couper notes that GHB is undetectable in the blood after only eight hours and in urine after 12 hours. Testing for it also requires a specific procedure, and with Rohypnol and related drugs, the dose typically used to facilitate sexual assaults can be undetectable.

College authorities fear the documented cases represent only a fraction of actual druggings.

Dr. Mary Watts, medical director of Hall Health Center on the UW campus, said she saw a sexual-assault victim within the last month who believed she had been drugged.

The girl said she had only one beer. Tests didn't show evidence of date-rape drugs, but that doesn't mean they weren't involved, Watts said.

The 22-year-old who experimented with GHB at her UW sorority house still wonders what would have happened if she hadn't been with friends.

"If I had gone to bed, I probably wouldn't have woken up," she said.

"I definitely think people need to know what it is and that it's out there. It's scary that it can just be put in someone's drink and given to anyone."

P-I reporter Ruth Schubert can be reached at 206-448-8130 or ruthschubert@seattle-pi.com
P-I reporter Kimberly A.C. Wilson contributed to this report.

behaviors, they may be diagnosed with an Anti-social Personality Disorder as they move into adulthood. As you will see in later in this chapter, when we discuss juvenile delinquency and the juvenile justice system, children who do not have empathy for others, frequently misinterpret the intentions of others towards them, and develop a

Table 12.7. Cardinal Signs and Symptoms: Conduct Disorder

- Aggressive to people and animals
- Bullies & initiates fights with others
- Has used a weapon
- Physically abused animals
- Sexually assaulted someone
- Steals directly from the victim
- Destruction of property and fire-setting
- Lying and theft
- Has entered someone's home & stolen
- Steals items with and without much value
- Runs away overnight
- Truancy from school

Table 12.8. Cardinal Signs and Symptoms: Oppositional Defiant Disorder

- Loses temper
- Argues with adults
- Refuses to follow rules
- Deliberately annoys others
- Blames others for mistakes
- Easily annoyed by others
- Angry and resentful
- Spiteful and vindictive

conduct disorder with sadistic behavior towards other people and pets, are at high risk to develop personality disorders. Table 12.7 describes the cardinal signs and symptoms of a child with Conduct Disorder while Table 12.8 describes the cardinal signs and symptoms of a child with Oppositional Defiant Disorder.

Eating Disorders

Eating disorders have become more commonly seen in children, particularly girls. They are usually diagnosed when the child does not maintain a normal minimum body weight (usually 85% of what is considered normal for the person's height), is afraid of gaining weight, and exhibits an unusual perception of his or her body image. The two most commonly diagnosed eating disorders are *anorexia nervosa*, which exists when the person fears gaining weight and refuses to eat and *bulimia*, which exists when the individual binges on food and then purges it by throwing up. These disorders can be very dangerous because those who have them have so altered their biochemical balance causing severe physiological illnesses and even death. For example, the popular singer Janis Joplin was said to have died from a chemical imbalance that caused her heart to stop as a result of an eating disorder. Residential treatment is usually needed to properly treat adolescents so that their food intake is carefully monitored, and whatever the psychological issues from their home that accompany this disorder can be dealt with without interference from the parental power struggles often seen with teenagers. There are some newer treatments that work with these youth in day treatment centers, but these are not common.

JUVENILE DELINQUENCY, STATUS CRIMES AND MENTAL DISORDERS

History

The history of the juvenile justice system began in 1899 with the first court that was especially started for juveniles established in Cook County (Chicago), Illinois. Within 30 years, all states had followed Chicago's lead and enacted laws and special rehabilitation services for responding to the needs of youth. It must be recognized that it wasn't until the late nineteenth century that youth were seen as different from miniature adults. At that time, a comprehensive mandatory public education system, child labor laws, and a child welfare system were developed to meet the state's responsibility for protecting youth. Children and youth were understood still to be in their formative years, so that personality could be more easily changed and shaped than when they became adults. Thus, their misconduct did not have to demonstrate that they would become hardened or *career criminals* as adults. In fact, today we have data that suggest that less than 20% of those arrested as youth will go on to become career criminals. This is amazing given the poor track record that we have in adequately providing for the needs of these youth.

Juvenile courts were by definition set up to be rehabilitative, not punitive or retributive. They were supposed to operate under the doctrine of *Parens Patriae*, which is the state serving as a wise and merciful substitute parent. It was seen as important to gain an understanding of children and their biopsychosocial needs. Rehabilitative decisions were to be made on the basis of what the child needed, not based on what acts the child had done to find himself or herself arrested. Thus, the sentencing decisions for a runaway girl (technically a status crime) might be the same as for a girl who was shoplifting (delinquent crime) if their needs were the same. Problems with this attitude began to emerge as the juvenile courts became overcrowded, resources to understand the youth became scarce, and violent crimes began to take center stage. Although violent crimes committed by juveniles actually have been decreasing over the past 15 years, the general public still believes that adolescents are very violent, and many people are afraid of them. The media attention on those crimes of violence committed by juveniles is responsible, at least in part, for this attitude.

In 1994, a Gallup poll indicated that Americans sampled believed that 43% of crime is due to juveniles while, in fact, only 13% of all crime is due to youth. However, although the number of juvenile crimes has decreased in general, the number of youth using guns to commit crimes doubled in the 5 year period between 1987 and 1992, and the number of violent crimes against persons by youth also increased by 56% during that time. So, although the overall crime rate is down, the violence used in crimes appears to be increasing. Even so, the number of teens murdered by adults is much higher than teens doing the killing. For example, six times as many teens are murdered by their parents than parents are murdered by teens. Over 70% of all teens who are killed are murdered by adults, not other youth. Obviously, the numbers of adults and teens killed during the rise in school violence in middle-class areas is also of concern, although school violence has been noted in inner city schools for decades.

Gender Issues

Offenses against persons by teens tend to be gender specific as they are with adults. In 1992, four out of every five violent offenses against other persons were committed by boys. Only 6% of violent offenses were reported committed by girls in 1992. Newer data from the Office of Juvenile Justice suggest that there is an increase in use of violence by girls at an even younger age. However, girls are more likely to engage in relational violence while boys are more likely to engage in gang violence, homicides and sexual offenses. Girls who are often depicted in popular media as angry and violent toward others are often suffering from PTSD from untreated trauma experienced in their own lives. This suggests that prevention of child abuse and intervention to alleviate PTSD could have a dramatic impact on lowering the aggressive behavior and violence used by both girls and boys. The prevalence of abuse in the backgrounds of girls arrested for violent crimes is often difficult to obtain in interviews as many of these girls minimize and deny that what has occurred is actually abuse. Recent research is presented in Box 12.5.

Children and Violent Crimes

Although anti-social and aggressive behavior can be noted at any age developmentally, if it develops earlier, when children are younger, it is more likely that the aggressive behavior will have persistence across the life span. In one study, 75% of those with a first arrest from 7 to 11 years old were found to be more likely to continue to a life of persistent use of violence and anti-social behavior. In fact, most of those children retrospectively were found to have conduct disorders as young as 3 years old.

BOX 12.5

Abuse Histories & PTSD Symptoms in Juvenile Girls

Juvenile girls have been presented as mean and angry when they commit violent acts against others. In trying to understand why they may be acting out in this way, research was conducted at Nova Southeastern University's Center for Psychological Studies and presented at the 2005 Annual Meeting of the American Psychological Association comparing the media portrayal of violent girls with the data obtained from girls who had been arrested and placed in a local juvenile detention center over a five-year period. It was found that the girls who were most likely to act out with aggression and violence were also those girls who had been exposed to the most trauma and had developed PTSD. Some of them were also demonstrating symptoms of depression. During interviews they minimized and denied the abuse they experienced but on standardized psychological measures that were administered, those who were the angriest were also the most traumatized. It was concluded that they were not "bad" girls who were simply looking for thrills as the movies like to sensationalize and portray them, but rather angry and traumatized young women, striking out of pain, not meanness. This is not to say they should not be held responsible for their behavior, but, rather, their rehabilitation rather than punishment must be a primary focus within the juvenile justice system. In fact, if they had been given the opportunity for treatment for PTSD earlier, their violent behavior might have been prevented.

This research was presented by Kendell Coker, Sonel Baute, Udak Ipke, Marva Robinson, & Lenore Walker in the symposium, Born to be Wild?, at the annual meeting of the American Psychological Association in Washington, D.C. in August 2005.

In comparison, only 25% of those youths who were arrested from ages 11 to 15 were found to continue their anti-social behavior through their life cycle. Interestingly, 80% of all youth in the juvenile justice system have no further arrests after age 21, and therefore, are assumed to have stopped their anti-social and aggressive behavior. However, it is unknown how many continue to physically or sexually abuse women and children in their families without being arrested.

Youth who end up using predatory violence (searching for victims outside of their homes) have certain characteristics consistent with later development of psychopathy, even though personality disorders are not completely formed until adulthood. This includes poor peer attachments and lack of empathy for the pain or other feelings of others. They are more prone to mood disorders, ADHD diagnoses, PTSD, Oppositional Defiant and Conduct Disorders, as well as neurological problems. Some symptoms of early onset child schizophrenia may occur as early as 15 to 16 years old, and as described earlier, these youth are prone to using drugs to self-medicate the symptomatology that they are unable to control in any other way. They are often noted to be rejected by peers as young as by the age of six. They have numerous school problems and their learning suffers.

Children who have been abused in their homes have been found to be at higher risk to use violence. In one study, risk was found to be 40%

higher than in non-abused children. In another study, boys who were exposed to violence in their homes were 700 times more likely to commit violence themselves. If they were also abused, which raised their risk to 1000 times those who have not been so exposed. Girls who use violence are even more likely to have been exposed to violence in their homes, especially early sexual victimization. As was described earlier, intervention programs for children exposed to domestic and street violence would go a long way to prevent the use of violence by both boys and girls.

Interestingly, youth who are more likely to become career criminals are more likely to misperceive intentions of other youth and adults towards them. In particular, they believe that people are behaving in a negative way towards them more often than is factually accurate. In some cases of violence, abusive men claim that they reacted quickly to feelings that they were disrespected. In addition to misperceiving aggressive intent, they are more likely to have problems in solving interpersonal conflict situations than others their age. This may be a result of the social rejection they typically experience as they are growing up. It is of critical importance to provide more corrective socialization experiences for at risk youth in order to prevent some of these lasting conditions.

Those who are mentally retarded make up a large proportion of the adult criminal population even though they are not as often arrested as youth. Youth with developmental delays or mental disorders who are in the wrong place at the wrong time may be easily coerced into confessing to crimes that they did not commit. Sometimes they may have been close enough to have seen what happened. Police have been known to take advantage of these youth when they want to solve a crime, especially if they already have a record of other delinquent behavior. In some rare cases, they are used by other delinquent youth in the community to commit crimes for the benefit of those delinquents. They may do so under duress, sometimes simply for friendship and promises of protection from harm, without actually understanding the nature and consequences of their behavior.

Again, it is important to remember that mental retardation has many causes that result in cognitive deficits, and these individuals probably act much younger than their chronological age. Interviewing techniques need to be tailored to the developmental level of the child's comprehension ability. These children may not be competent to understand what has happened or what will happen to them after an arrest. They may not have the requisite mental capability to predict that something bad will happen even if they hear discussions between others. The number of youth arrested who are not competent to understand their Miranda rights, including the right to have a parent and an attorney present when being questioned by law enforcement or to stop the questioning at any time, is astounding.

BOX 12.6
MacArthur Competency Standards

Understanding of charges and potential consequences

1. Ability to understand and appreciate the charges and their seriousness.
2. Ability to understand possible dispositional consequences of guilty, not guilty, and not guilty by reason of insanity.
3. Ability to realistically appraise the likely outcomes.

Understanding of the trial process

4. Ability to understand, without significant distortion, the roles of participants in the trial process (ie: judge, defense attorney, witness, jury).
5. Ability to understand the process and potential consequences of pleading and plea bargaining.

6. Ability to grasp the general sequence of pretrial and trial events.

Capacity to Participate with Attorney in a Defense

7. Ability to adequately trust or work collaboratively with attorney.
8. Ability to disclose to attorney reasonably coherent description of facts pertaining to charges, as perceived by the defendant.
9. Ability to reason about available options by weighing their consequences, without significant distortion.
10. **Potential for Courtroom Participation** Ability to testify coherently, if testimony is needed.
11. Ability to control own behavior during trial proceedings.
12. Ability to manage the stress of trial.

Competency to Waive Miranda and Stand Trial

Competency is a legal term that has been defined by state legislatures to mean that someone possesses the *mens rea* or a guilty or culpable mind that intended the crime to happen and is sufficiently able to comprehend the legal proceedings in which he or she is involved. This is part of the British common law system that the U.S. has adapted. Assessment of the ability to think and comprehend information is part of the forensic psychologist's job. When assessing for competency, it is important to understand how the emotional state of the person impacts on his or her ability to think, make good judgments, and comprehend what was in the past, is presently, and will in the future occur. For children, this means assessing developmental ability as well as thoughts and emotions as they impact on behavior and cognition. Many children do not have the requisite mental ability because of the social conditions in which they live, usually including poverty, poor nutrition, violence in their homes, and on the streets within their communities.

Children may be able to describe, by rote, the roles of the people in the justice system without actually comprehending how it all works in sufficient detail to assist their attorney in defending themselves. Psychologist Thomas Grisso has developed a psychological assessment instrument to measure competency in youth that is consistent with most of the statutes on competency in effect today. The MacArthur Foundation has funded a study of how to assess for competency in adults and youth. The important areas to assess when measuring children's competency can be found in Box 12.6. Although there are other competency tests for children, in using them, fewer than 15% of those arrested for delinquency are found not to be competent. However, the

---

BOX 12.7

Lional Tate Case

Florida, interestingly, has no requirement for a waiver hearing. Rather, any youth can be charged with a serious crime by the prosecutor and automatically waived into adult court, and the judge or defense has no choice in the matter. Judges are permitted to take the youth's age into account, but they are not required to do so. Sometimes the psychologists' findings are admitted into testimony, but it is not uncommon for two psychologists to come to different opinions, often because they have different sources of data. Competency may change from day to day or even hour to hour, especially in seriously mentally ill youth. Sometimes, a mentally ill youth, usually an adolescent, may also be very manipulative and tell different stories to different people. Two cases have attracted national attention to Florida in this area: Broward County's Lionel Tate, who admitted wrestling a 6 year old girl whom his mother was babysitting, to death, when he was 12 years old, and Nathaniel Brazil, a 14 year old West Palm Beach youth who shot and killed his teacher after being angry because he was sent him home from school.

Tate, whose mother convinced him to turn down a plea agreement with a three year sentence was convicted, becoming the youngest person in the United States sentenced to spend the rest of his life in prison. Nathaniel Brazil was found guilty of manslaughter and received a much lighter sentence than would an adult. Why the differences? One reason might have been the discrepant opinions offered by psychologists on the witness stand about mental competency at different developmental ages. Another possible reason might have been Tate's behavior—he had a long history of aggressive behavior and was noted to be a violent and disturbed child at an early age.

After three years in adult confinement, the Florida appellate court granted Tate a new trial, in part, because the court claimed the original psychologist did not do a thorough competency examination. Under a plea arrangement, he was released with credit for the time he served in prison and placed on probation. However, the damage was already done, and he has been back in custody awaiting trial for a violation of his probation as well as for armed robbery, unable to stay out of trouble with the law. Interestingly, his attorney attempted to get him to accept a plea to the new charges but Tate shortly afterwards wrote to the judge saying he did not understand the consequences of the long prison sentence when he accepted that plea. The judge has ordered new competency evaluations so his fate is still unknown. How much damage had already been done prior to incarceration with adult criminals and how much further emotional damage came from his identification with other criminals has yet to be assessed, if possible.

MacArthur studies strongly suggest that competency be determined only after multiple data sources are examined, including prior arrest history, presence of mental retardation or borderline intelligence, interviews with parents or juvenile authorities who know the child, history of mental illness, history of conduct disorder and school records. The arrest report, probable cause affidavit, and statement of witnesses should also be available. In addition, special attention should be paid to language issues, cultural context, passivity, ability to acquiesce to authority persons, and ability to be confused. Box 12.7 provides an outline of the factors that the MacArthur studies have found relevant.

Waiver to Adult Court

There are three major ways that youth may be diverted from the juvenile system: dismissal of the charges if already charged, civil commitment to psychiatric care, and automatic *waiver* to adult criminal court. Juveniles who commit serious crimes may be charged as an adult and tried and punished there. The law accepts that a youth who kills or rapes someone needs to be held responsible for her or his actions and the burden to prove that he or she is not mentally competent or responsible is on the youth. In most states, a hearing may be requested to determine the mental status of the youth for whom a waiver into adult court is requested, usually if the youth is over 14 years old. Psychologists often conduct clinical interviews, administer standardized psychological tests, and offer testimony at these hearings. Although the decisions should be based on the youth's competency and ability to be held responsible for his or her behavior; in fact, the type of acts committed and prior criminal history are often given more weight than the psychologist's findings.

It is important to think about goals when punishing youth for their behavior. If indeed rehabilitation is the goal, then placing children with other youth who have emotional problems and have committed bad acts, will only enhance the possibility that these youth will continue in a life of adult crime. Learning theory is pretty clear; children repeat the behavior for which they get social attention. They learn most from their peers as adolescents. If they are placed with other peers who have problems with behavioral control, such as occurs in so-called *boot camps*, they are more likely to learn more bad behavior. If they are placed with other peers with good behavior, and they are rewarded with attention focused on their good behavior, they are most likely to change their negativity and aggression. This may be an important reason why boot camps have been unsuccessful in preventing recidivism.

Those with active psychotic symptoms are the most likely to be violent, especially if they are experiencing delusions or hallucinations. It is important for law enforcement officers to understand that, if they are approaching a teen who may be in a psychotic or drug induced psychotic-like state, they must use non-aggressive and carefully chosen means of making contact with the youth so as to avoid setting off a violent incident. If these youth are more likely to misperceive aggressive intent on the part of a law enforcement officer, it may also be a good idea to approach in an overly friendly manner so that the officer's intentions are made very clear from the outset. This is often counter-intuitive because many believe that it is important to establish who is "boss" right from the start. However, there are many techniques that can be used to remain firm, but friendly and non-aggressive, to avoid any misperceptions and unnecessary force when dealing with these youth.

School Violence

Children who commit violence in the schools are becoming more easily identified because other children are feeling more secure in reporting them as bullies. However, some of those who committed serial killings inside school, such as those involved in the Columbine High School

---

BOX 12.8

School Violence Risk Investigation Model

Category 1

High Violence Potential—Imminent Risk for Harm
Qualifies for immediate hospitalization or arrest

Category 2

High Violence Potential—High Risk for Harm
Needs Services as has High Risk Warning Signs
Physical altercation with another person
Frequent fights
Inappropriate weapons use or possession
Drawings or other creative outlets with persistent violent themes
Attire associated with violence (ie, camouflage fatigues, violent messages on t-shirts
Physically intimidates peers and younger children.
Following/surveilling target individuals
Short fused, loss of emotional control
Destruction of property
Bullying or victim of bullying
Deteriorating physical appearance
Violent literature and hate group materials
Inappropriate displays of emotion including anger, hate, rage, depression
Isolating and withdrawn
Signs of or history of substance use/abuse/dependency
Signs of depression/severe mood swings
Rebellion against school authority
Identifiable violent taboos

Category 3

Insufficient Evidence Potential—Moderate Risk for Harm

Potential Evidence Repetitive & Intentional Emotional Distress
Has high risk signs and some stabilizing factors

Category 4

Insufficient Evidence of Violence—Minor Risk for Harm
Potential Evidence Unintentional Emotional Distress
Insensitive and some warning & stabilizing signs
Self as victim of a particular person
Grudges & deep resentments
Particular object of desire including unrequited love turned to hate, shame, rage, etc.
Perceived injustices, humiliation & disrespect
Thoughts of death and violence
Narrow focus—no way out—tunnel vision
Aggression immersion
    Theme is consistent
    Sequence specific stimulation
Publicized acts of violence
Historically violent figures
Violent music and other media
Weapons & destruction
Stalking
    Simple obsessional
    Love obsessional
    Erotomania

Category 5

Insufficiency Evidence of Violence—Low Risk for Harm
Insufficient Evidence for Emotional Distress
Misunderstandings, peer trouble & poor decisions

This information is taken from Kris Mohandie (2000). Threat Assessment in Schools. Specialized Training: San Diego, CA.

---

massacre in Littleton, Colorado in April 1999, were considered more odd than bullies. There are numerous incidents where youth physically and psychologically bully and hurt others daily. Interestingly, all those who engaged in reported school massacres were boys. However, as was described earlier, high school age girls are violent towards each other and others also. Psychologists Chris Hatcher and Kris Mohandie set forth some guidelines for assessment of risk of school violence for anyone working with schools to insure that they protect other children, faculty, and staff from further violence by these youth. These guidelines can be found in Box 12.8.

Finally, we have attempted to demonstrate how intertwined the mental health, biological fitness, and life experiences of youth will impact on their behavior in crisis situations and in the commission of juvenile crimes. There are numerous resources that can be of assistance when attempting to intervene and rehabilitate children no matter how destructive their behavior or how hopeless it seems. Many of the attempts that have been set up by society, to assist these youth who come to our attention, such as detention centers, boot camps, foster family care, residential treatment centers, teen drug courts and mental health centers appear to be based on good theory and intentions but they are not very effective. Most of the time it is because funding is inadequate to carry out the entire program, so only parts of it are implemented. Often politics gets in the way especially when multicultural issues are in the forefront. The Gains Center (www.gainsctr.com) operates a resource center designed to assist communities that are trying out new programs. It will be important for the community to make decisions whether adolescent offenders will be treated as adults or juveniles if we can save more youth from moving ahead into career criminal paths.

SUGGESTED READINGS

Barry, K. (1979). *Female sexual slavery*. New York: NYU Press.

Carll, E. K. (1999). *Violence in our lives: Impact on workplace, home & community*. Needham, MA: Allyn & Bacon.

Courtois, C. A. (1999). *Recollections of sexual abuse: Treatment principles & Guidelines*. New York: Norton.

Evans, D. L., Foa, E. B., Gur, R. E., Hendin, H., O'Brien, C. P., Seligman, M. E. P., & Walsh, B. T. (2005). *Treating and preventing adolescent mental health disorders*. New York: Oxford.

Erez, E. & Laster, K. (Ed.). (2000). *Domestic violence: Global responses*. Oxfordshire, England: A.B. Academic Publishers.

Herman, J. L. (1992). *Trauma and recovery*. New York: Basic Books.

Koss, M. P., Goodman, L. A., Browne, A., Fitzgerald, L. F., Keita, G., & Russo, N. F. (1994). *No safe haven: Male violence of women at home, at work, and in the Community*. Washington, DC: American Psychological Associaton.

Kuehnle, K. (1996). *Assessing allegations of child sexual abuse*. Sarasota, FL: Professional Resources Press.

La Grecca, A. M., Sevin, S. W., & Sevin, E. L. (2005). *After the storm: A guide to help children cope with the psychological effects of a hurricane*. Coral Gables, FL: 7-Dippity, Inc.

Meloy, J. R. (Ed.). (1998). *The psychology of stalking*. New York: Academic Press.

Mohandie, K. (2002). Human captivity experiences. *Journal of Threat Assessment, 2.*

Mohandie, K., Meloy, J. R., McGowan, M. G., & Williams, J. (2006). The RECON Typology of stalking: Reliability and validity based upon a large sample of North American stalkers. *Journal of Forensic Science, 51,* 147–155.

Peled, E., Jaffe, P. G., & Edelman, J. L. (Eds.). (1995). *The cycle of violence: Community Responses to children of battered women.* Thousand Oaks, CA: Sage.

Perry, G. P. & Orchard, J. (1992). *Assessment and treatment of adolescent sex offenders.* Sarasota, FL: Professional Resources Press.

Walker, L. E. A. (2000). *The Battered Woman Syndrome Second Edition.* New York: Springer.

Walker, L. E. A. (1994). *Abused women and Survivor Therapy: A practical guide for the Psychotherapist.* Washington, DC: American Psychological Association.

Index